The Effectiveness of Medical Care

The Johns Hopkins Series in Contemporary Medicine and Public Health

Consulting Editors
Samuel H. Boyer IV, M.D.
Gareth M. Green, M.D., M.P.H.
Richard T. Johnson, M.D.
Paul R. McHugh, M.D.
Edmond A. Murphy, M.D.
Albert H. Owens, Jr., M.D.
Jerry L. Spivak, M.D.
Barbara Starfield, M.D., M.P.H.

The Effectiveness of Medical Care: Validating Clinical Wisdom

Barbara Starfield, M.D., M.P.H.

with
Lisa Egbuonu, M.D., M.P.H.
Mark Farfel
Nancy Hutton, M.D.
Alain Joffe, M.D., M.P.H.
Lawrence S. Wissow, M.D.

The Johns Hopkins University Press
Baltimore and London

© 1985 The Johns Hopkins University Press
All rights reserved
Printed in the United States of America

The Johns Hopkins University Press, 701 West 40th Street,
Baltimore, Maryland 21211
The Johns Hopkins Press Ltd, London

The paper in this book is acid-free and meets the
guidelines for permanence and durability of the
Committee on Production Guidelines for Book Longevity
of the Council on Library Resources.

Library of Congress Cataloging in Publication Data

Starfield, Barbara.
   The effectiveness of medical care.

  (The Johns Hopkins series in contemporary medicine
and public health)
   Includes bibliographies and index.
   1. Children—Diseases—Treatment—Evaluation.
I. Title. II. Series. [DNLM: 1. Quality of Health
Care. 2. Therapeutics—infancy & childhood.
WS 366 S7945e]
RJ52.S83 1985   362.1′9892   84-21807
ISBN 0-8018-3260-8

This book is dedicated with unbounded love to my parents, Eva and Martin Starfield, teachers par excellence, role models without equal.

Contents

List of Figures xi
List of Tables xiii
Foreword by Frederick C. Robbins, M.D. xv
Acknowledgments xvii

1. Introduction 1

Part I. Child Health Problems Amenable to Prevention by Medical Care through Reduction in the Frequency of Occurrence
2. Neonatal Mortality 9
3. Postneonatal Mortality 20
4. Low Birth Weight 24
5. Teenage Childbearing 37
6. Inadequate Immunizations and the Prevention of Communicable Diseases 48
7. Acute Rheumatic Fever 58
8. Child Battering (Abuse) 63

Part II. Child Health Problems Amenable to Prevention by Medical Care through Detection and Management in the Premorbid Stage
9. Congenital Hypothyroidism and Phenylketonuria 71
10. Lead Poisoning 76
11. Iron-Deficiency Anemia 87

Part III. Child Health Problems Amenable to Treatment by Medical Care through Prevention of Complications or Sequelae
12. Diabetes: Prevention of Ketoacidosis 97
13. Convulsive Disorders (Epilepsy): Prevention of Status Epilepticus 103
14. Bacterial Meningitis: Prevention of Sequelae 109

15. Acute Appendicitis: Prevention of Complications   120
16. Asthma   130
17. Gastroenteritis and Dehydration   136

Part IV. Caveats, Considerations, and Conclusions
18. The Findings in Perspective   145

Notes on Contributors   161
Index   163

Figures

1. Fetal and Infant Mortality, United States, 1940–83   10
2. Neonatal Mortality Rates in New York City by Ethnic Group, 1950–71   11
3. Percentage Decline in Infant Mortality, 1915–80   21
4. Incidence of Prematurity in New York City by Ethnic Group, 1955–71   28
5. Percentage of Women Who Have Borne One or More Children by Age 17, by Race, United States, 1917–78   40
6. Reported Cases of Poliomyelitis (Paralytic), United States, 1951–81   49
7. Reported Cases of Measles (Rubeola), United States, 1955–81   50
8. Reported Cases of Pertussis (Whooping Cough) and Deaths, United States, 1922–81   51
9. Reported Cases of Rubella (German Measles), United States, 1966–81   52
10. Measles Cases and Federal Grant Funds Obligated for Measles Control Programs, United States, 1965–76   55
11. Incidence of Rheumatic Fever in Four Studies: Malmö, Sweden; Connecticut; Rochester, Minnesota; and Nashville, Tennessee   59
12. Incidence of Epilepsy in Rochester Study   104

Tables

1. Percentage of Infants Weighing 2,500 Grams or Less at Birth, United States, 1950–64   26
2. Percentage of Infants Weighing 2,500 Grams or Less at Birth, United States, 1965–79   27
3. Selected Natality Indicators for Women under 20, United States, 1950–80   38
4. Summary of Studies Reporting Prevalence of Iron-Deficiency Anemia in Young Children, 1932–74   88
5. Age-Specific Incidence of Reported Bacterial Meningitis, United States, 1978   110
6. Incidence Ratio and Survival for Patients with Str. Pneumoniae, N. Meningitidis, and H. Influenzae Meningitis, Boston City Hospital, 1935–72   114
7. Annual Incidence and Rates of Appendicitis in Children Less Than 15 Years, United States, 1968, 1971, 1972, 1978, and 1979   121
8. Deaths in Children Due to Appendicitis, United States, 1950–78   123
9. Death Rates in Children Due to Appendicitis, United States, 1950–78   124
10. Percentage with Appendiceal Perforation by Age   125
11. Average Length of Hospital Stay for Acute Appendicitis in Children with and without Perforation   126
12. Percentage of Appendicitis Cases with Perforation, by Family Income, Huntington, West Virginia, 1976–78   127

Foreword

It is only within recent times that serious questions have been asked about the effectiveness of medical treatments and procedures. Traditionally, physicians relied upon clinical judgment that came with experience in order to assess the value of what they did. Needless to say, this rarely involved much in the way of systematic evaluation that would stand the test of statistical validity. In the last thirty to forty years the randomized clinical trial (RCT) has been employed to assess efficacy and has become recognized as one of the soundest evaluation strategies available. For a variety of reasons, including their cost, ethical considerations, and difficulties in conducting them, RCTs have been applied to relatively few technologies. Furthermore, RCTs measure efficacy and effectiveness. Means such as retrospective analyses, the use of registries for the systematic accumulation of data over time, and the analysis of vital statistics or data obtained from surveys such as the National Health Examination Survey conducted by the National Center for Health Statistics have been employed to make some estimates of effectiveness; these vary greatly in their precision, however. The fact of the matter is that we still engage in many practices in medical care that have not been subjected to formal assessment nor indeed are we as systematic as we might be in evaluating new technologies. However, as more and more technologies are developed and introduced into the marketplace and with the steadily mounting pressure to control costs it becomes important, over and above the issue of safety, to discourage the use of ineffective technologies and to encourage those that are both effective and, best of all, cost effective. Making such determinations, of course, requires some way of measuring outcome, which in and of itself is often difficult. Medical outcomes themselves are often hard to quantify; personal, psychological, and social outcomes are even more elusive.

Dr. Starfield has reviewed the evidence for the effectiveness of medical care in improving outcomes in a number of medical conditions. It is important to recognize that Dr. Starfield has undertaken a difficult task because often she is analyzing the effectiveness of a system of care the components of which cannot easily be analyzed individually (e.g., neonatal mortality, low birth weight, and the impact of prenatal care), in contrast to the evaluation of a drug or single procedure (e.g., immunization or congenital hypothyroidism). Furthermore, when one attempts to analyze effectiveness as opposed to efficacy, the various practical factors involved in providing a satisfactory delivery system influence the outcome in a manner that cannot be controlled neatly.

The results of Dr. Starfield's analysis are important from two distinct points of view. First, she presents convincing evidence for the effectiveness of medical care in a number of important conditions of childhood. One might respond that this is belaboring the obvious, we knew that all the time. However, in some of the conditions that she examines there has been much discussion about the role of medical care as opposed to the role of altered social circumstances, e.g., as in the case of teenage pregnancies. Second, one cannot help but be impressed by the relatively few data there are that can be used for the kind of analysis done by Dr. Starfield and how questionably reliable even they are. Indeed, in some instances, such as assessing the value of that long-established ritual of childhood, removal of the tonsils and adenoids, adequate data are still not in hand and it is only recently that any systematic evaluations have been attempted.

Thus, it is somewhat reassuring to find that medical care is of value in many childhood conditions, but dismaying to realize how sparse are the data relevant to this issue and that many of the things that we do in medical care have never been satisfactorily documented as effective.

If we are to develop a health care system that is as effective as possible, we will have to develop better methods than exist now to assess and monitor the impact of medical care on a range of health problems. Dr. Starfield's analysis serves an important function in summarizing what is known and, perhaps more important, highlighting needs for the future.

Frederick C. Robbins, M.D.
President, Institute of Medicine
National Academy of Sciences

Acknowledgments

Encouragement and partial financial support for the review of evidence were provided by the Robert Wood Johnson Foundation. (The views expressed in this book are those of the authors and no official endorsement by the Robert Wood Johnson Foundation is intended or should be inferred.) The book was completed while the author was a Henry J. Kaiser Senior Fellow at the Center for Advanced Study in the Behavioral Sciences.

At the time the review was conducted, Nancy Hutton was a Fellow in the Robert Wood Johnson Foundation General Pediatric Academic Training Program, Lawrence S. Wissow was a Mellon Fellow in Clinical Epidemiology, and Mark Farfel was receiving support from the National Center for Health Services Research in the doctoral program of the Department of Health Policy and Management, all at the Johns Hopkins University Medical Institutions.

The authors are grateful for the suggestions and help provided by the following individuals in the identification of sources for the data in the monograph.

Adolescent Childbearing
  Anne Duggan, B.A.
  Lorraine Klerman, Dr. P.H.
  Constance Nathanson, Ph.D.
  Laurie Zabin, Sc.D.
Inadequate Immunization and
  Contagious Diseases
  Alan Hinman, M.D., M.P.H.
  Camara Jones, M.D., M.P.H.
  Marshall McBean, M.D., M.P.H.
Hypothyroidism and
  Phenylketonuria
  Neil A. Holtzman, M.D.
Gastroenteritis and Dehydration
  Mathuram Santosham, M.D.
Asthma
  Peyton Eggleston, M.D.

Appendicitis
  David Dudgeon, M.D.
  Mark Ravitch, M.D.
Bacterial Meningitis
  Leighton E. Cluff, M.D.
  Ralph Feigin, M.D.
  Roger Feldman, M.D.
  David Fraser, M.D.
  Edward Mortimer, M.D.
  Richard Moxon, M.D.
  Gary Overturf, M.D.
Diabetes
  Nina Berlin
  John Davidson, M.D.
  Allan Drash, M.D.
  Donald Etzwiler, M.D.
  Howard Fishbein, M.D.

Ray Kuehne
Leona Miller, M.D.
Leslie Plotnick, M.D.
Arlan Rosenbloom, M.D.
Chris Saudek, M.D.
Pomeroy Sinnick, M.D.
Leslie Waldman
Fred Whitehouse, M.D.
T. Franklin Williams, M.D.

Epilepsy
John Freeman, M.D.
Daniel Shapiro (National Epilepsy Library)

Iron-Deficiency Anemia
Robert Drachman, M.D.
Modena Wilson, M.D.

Acute Rheumatic Fever
Leon Gordis, M.D., Dr. P.H.
Robert Pantell, M.D.

Child Battering
Linda Heisner
Lewis Margolis, M.D.

For initial judgments leading to selection of conditions
Susan Brink, MSHA
Peter Budetti, M.D., J.D.
Marie C. McCormick, M.D., Sc.D.
Alvin Novack, M.D.
Robert Pantell, M.D.
Frederick Rivara, M.D.
Modena Wilson, M.D., M.P.H.

The author is also grateful to Diane Rowland, M.P.A., and George Silver, M.D., for their insightful comments and helpful suggestions.

The Effectiveness of Medical Care

1
Introduction

Barbara Starfield

Why bother to document the benefits of medical care? After all, people continue to seek care when they perceive a need for it; an educated population accustomed to expecting value in commodities would certainly reject a product that consistently failed to achieve its promise. Many people continue to believe in the benefits of medical care. Others, however, maintain that such care has little demonstrable impact. Moreover, the medical literature generally fails to address directly the issue of effectiveness. The purpose of this book is to draw together information that is widely scattered, and systematically to explore the nature of the evidence as it pertains to important conditions affecting the health of children.

Relentlessly increasing costs of health services rather than doubts about effectiveness have been responsible for the popularity of the view that medical care is an oversold commodity. But the rising costs of care have not been the only reason for the concerns. Some thoughtful analysts conclude that medical care has little to offer as an approach to improving the health of the public, particularly when compared to the contribution of social and nutritional advances (McKeown 1979). Others argue cogently about the limitations of modern medicine (Powles 1973) and for alternative approaches to ill health (Carlson 1975). There are even some who consider medical care detrimental to health (Illich 1976) and some who claim that further improvements in morbidity rates will result only if individuals alter their styles of living (Lalonde 1974). Doubts are so prevalent that sporadic evidence concerning reductions in the frequency of specific conditions after development of improved medical technology (McDermott 1978; Rogers, Blendon, Moloney 1982) and systematic attempts to show the relative merits of late and early interventions for the treatment and management of health problems seem to have had little impact.

Economic pressures to reduce expenditures for medical care make the question more than an academic one. Lack of evidence of beneficial results provides a convenient excuse to withdraw financing for some types of services, particularly where they are perceived as a drain on public funds. Clinical wisdom is no longer a sufficient argument. In fact, the stimulus for this review was concern that the possibility of impending cutbacks in publicly financed services would jeopardize the health of children. Some professional groups, the Ambulatory Pediatric Association in particular, organized task forces to document the impact of these changes in public policy, but the search for appropriate measures of impact was compromised by the unavailability of concrete evidence of the benefits of medical care for children. Other impending changes in organization and financing raise equally important questions regarding the value of medical care.

How can we be reasonably sure that medical care for children has been fulfilling its assumed purpose, at least most of the time? Three assumptions guided the approach taken in this book: (1) that the argument is best made using information concerning relatively common conditions; (2) that indirect measures of effectiveness of care can substitute for direct measures when the latter are unavailable; and (3) that the major benefits of medical care can be expected for prevention and early rather than late intervention in the process of disease (Holtzman 1979). The following section describes how these assumptions guided the approach.

Methods of Selecting Conditions and Assessing Benefits

The initial list of conditions was derived from the "sentinel" problems as reported by Rutstein et al. (1976). These problems should be preventable with current medical interventions. Some conditions, however, were not further considered because they were infrequent. Others were eliminated because their occurrence is associated primarily with poor or unjustified medical practices (as is frequently the case for tonsillectomy and adenoidectomy) or is a consequence of the failure of medical personnel to perform indicated procedures (such as case-finding among contacts of teenagers with venereal disease). The effort, therefore, was to assess the value of access to and receipt of medical care rather than to determine the usefulness of particular medical interventions. Six pediatric experts provided their ratings (on a scale of 0–3) of the extent to which each of the remaining 27 conditions would be affected by removal of specific medical programs or changes in financing of services (such as decreased reimbursements or institution of copayments for services). Although there was substantial variability in judgments for many of the conditions, the conditions chosen for review represent those that are relatively common and those for which there was consensus that medical care is important.

The indirect measures of effectiveness were of three types. The first of these involved changes in the frequency of mortality or morbidity consequent to changes in financing or organization of services. As such changes in the health system were particularly notable following legislation in the mid and late 1960s to institute programs such as Medicaid and community health centers, longitudinal trends in morbidity and mortality across that time period provide much information of the first type. The second type of evidence concerned inferences about health or illness in population groups thought to be at least relatively deprived of medical care. For example, higher illness rates of people living in remote geographic areas might be considered indirect evidence of the benefit of medical care because the individuals are known to have difficulty in getting to a source of care and no other explanation for greater illness is found. Similarly, higher illness rates of people who are unable to afford care could be considered indirect evidence of effectiveness if there is no other plausible explanation. The third approach involved clinical data concerning the occurrence of complications or sequelae of illness consequent to delay in receiving medical care.

The benefits expected from medical care were of three types: reduction in the frequency of occurrence of the condition; detection of the condition in its early (pre-morbid) stage; and prevention of complications or sequelae of the condition. Conditions primarily amenable to prevention of occurrence or reduction in frequency of occurrence were neonatal mortality, postneonatal mortality, low birth weight, teenage childbearing, inadequate immunization and the communicable diseases, acute rheumatic fever, and child battering. (Child battering originally was placed with the third category but review of the evidence on effectiveness of care was responsible for its movement to the first category.) Conditions in the second category were congenital hypothyroidism and phenylketonuria, lead poisoning, and iron deficiency anemia. The third category included most approaches to diabetes, epilepsy, bacterial meningitis, acute appendicitis, asthma, and gastroenteritis.

In reviewing the evidence, only studies of the effect of medical care as generally practiced were included. That is, studies of efficacy alone were not considered as sources of information on effectiveness. However, an attempt was made to provide at least a theoretical justification for expecting medical care to be beneficial, and where actual evidence was available, it is cited. Demonstration projects that have not been widely adopted or studies of unusual or novel types of care were not considered to have provided sufficiently definitive evidence to warrant their being included. Although these studies may have significant implications for how medical care *should* be provided, they do not adequately represent the way in which medical care *is* generally provided at the current time, at least in the United States.

Several other criteria guided the selection of studies for inclusion. Data concerning adults alone were not included where information pertaining specifically to children was available. Where national data were available, these received priority over local or regional data. Moreover, studies of whole communities were selected in preference to studies in particular institutions. That is, emphasis was placed on epidemiologic studies and on studies from more than one area. Where studies using superior research design and better research methods were available, studies with relatively poor or inadequate design were not cited. With rare exception (when few other data were available) only published studies were used. Both computerized literature searches and personal consultation with a wide network of experts in each field were used to identify relevant studies. Special emphasis was placed on studies employing control or comparison groups. Relatively recent studies were cited in preference to older studies, unless these were useful in assessing the beneficial effects of changes in medical care delivery. This principle was followed in order to avoid drawing conclusions based upon outdated medical technology.

Differences in the amount of data in the following chapters are a reflection primarily of differences in the extent to which subjects have received the attention of researchers. This is probably due, at least in part, to the availability of data for analysis. In particular, there appear to be fewer data for conditions where the sources of information are clinical facilities, as compared with data collected by federal or local efforts mandated by law. In all cases, however, an attempt was made to follow the same outline in each of the chapters: a first section that addresses the incidence and/or prevalence of the condition; the impact of the condition (except for the chapters on mortality); and a summary of the basis for expecting that medical care would be effective; and a second section presenting evidence regarding effectiveness.

Evaluating the effectiveness of current medical care is a difficult and perhaps often impossible task. In situations where therapy is well established by custom, ethical considerations preclude experimentation. Even if ethical problems were resolved, attempts to mount controlled clinical trials would quickly overtax the supply of qualified investigators and available research funds. Even if it were possible, however, it is unlikely to be the most prudent approach. Controlled clinical trials provide evidence of efficacy. That is, they indicate whether a procedure or therapy works as it is intended to work when the conditions of its application are specified and generally as optimal as possible. In contrast, most therapies in practice cannot be applied under pre-specified conditions. It is usually not possible to ensure that people will perform the prescribed regimen exactly as directed, and potential inhibitory effects stemming from the exigencies of everyday life cannot be anticipated, much less checked. Studies that examine the effectiveness of medical care, that is, its impact under conditions that more nearly simulate ordinary reality, are few and far between. Retrospective evaluations, such as most of those cited in the following pages, have their own limitations. They cannot be based on random allocation of subjects and it is never possible to be sure that comparison groups are equivalent to study groups with regard to factors that may be of greatest importance. It is also possible that those studies failing to confirm the suspicions of the investigators are less likely to be published than results of prospective trials, and this may lead to a bias favoring studies showing that medical care is effective.

With all of these caveats, the following review of the effectiveness of medical care for these conditions reflects the state of affairs as of the late 1970s and early 1980s in the United States.

References

Carlson R. The end of medicine. New York: John Wiley & Sons, 1975.

Holtzman N. Prevention: rhetoric and reality. Int J Health Serv 1979;8:25-9.

Illich I. Medical nemesis: the expropriation of health. New York: Pantheon Books, 1976.

Lalonde M. A new perspective in the health of Canadians. Ottawa: Government of Canada, 1974.

McDermott W. Medicine: the public good and one's own. Persp Biol Med 1978;21:167-87.

McKeown T. The role of medicine: dream, mirage, or nemesis? Princeton, N.J.: Princeton Univ Press, 1979.

Powles J. On the limitations of modern medicine. Sci Med Man 1973;1:1-30.

Rogers D, Blendon R, Moloney T. Who needs Medicaid? N Engl J Med 1982;307;13-18.

Rutstein D, Berenberg W, Chalmers T, Child C, Fishman A, Perrin E. Measuring the quality of medical care: a clinical method. N Engl J Med 1976;294:582-88 (tables revised May 1980).

Part I

Child Health Problems Amenable to Prevention by Medical Care through Reduction in the Frequency of Occurrence

2
Neonatal Mortality

Barbara Starfield

Of all relatively common medical problems, it is perhaps easiest to document the effectiveness of medical care in reducing neonatal mortality (deaths in the first 27 days of life). Moreover, evidence comes from a variety of sources. This chapter reviews the nature of the evidence from both retrospective and prospective approaches. As the body of literature is vast, and of uneven quality, no attempt has been made to review all or even most of the published studies. Only studies thought to be the best of their kind are cited. Since the focus of the review is the effectiveness of medical care, the large number of studies concerning only the influence of sociodemographic factors are not cited. In most cases, the most important of these variables are included as control variables in the best studies of the effectiveness of medical care. Where possible, evidence regarding disparities between neonatal mortality rates (NMR) of poor and nonpoor populations are also addressed.

In the 15 years between 1950 and 1965 neonatal mortality in the United States declined only slightly (see Figure 1). In some areas, neonatal mortality increased. Figure 2, from Pakter and Nelson (1974), provides data from New York City and shows the extent to which neonatal mortality rose, particularly among nonwhite infants. Nationwide, there was no improvement in neonatal survival in any of the low birth weight groups (2,500 grams or less), who are at highest risk of death, and only slight improvement at "normal" birth weights (over 2,500 grams). The gap in neonatal mortality between white and black infants widened (Shapiro et al. 1968, 14). This markedly slowed decline in the rate of fall of NMR has been attributed to an increase in teenage pregnancies, a trend toward greater poverty, and movement of large segments of the population from rural areas with a consequent increase in registration of births and deaths. It is certain that the trend nationwide was not due to an increase in nonwhite births (which account for only a small proportion of the trend) or to an increase in the proportion of

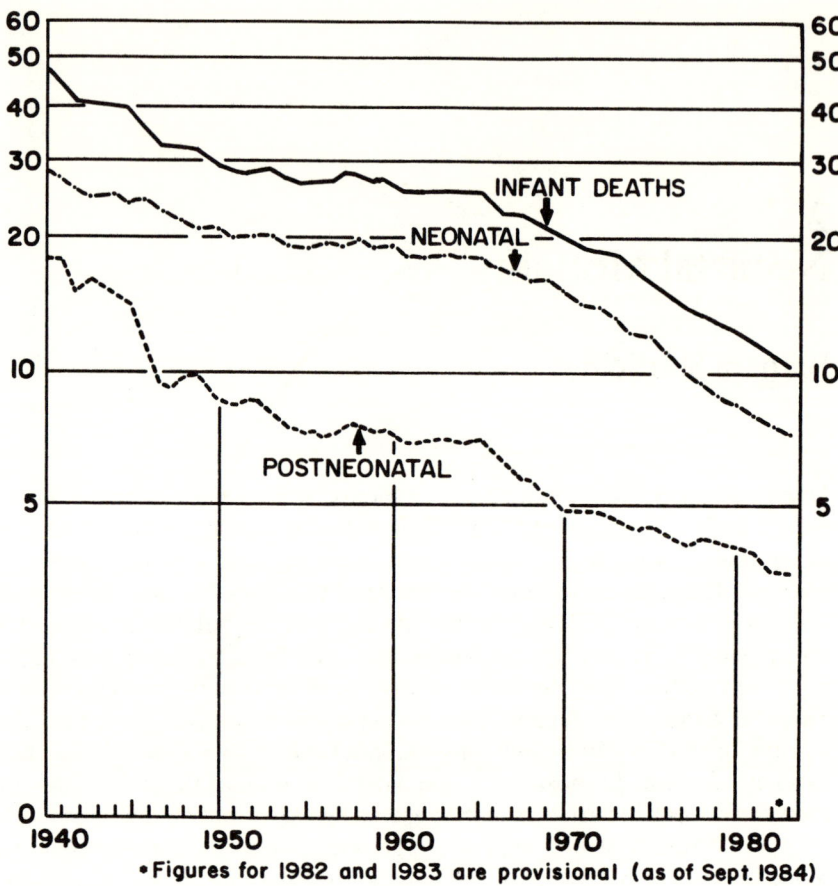

Figure 1. Fetal and Infant Mortality, United States, 1940–83
Source: NCHS, Vital Statistics of the United States, annual volumes.

infants born at low birth weights. As a result of their extensive analysis of the problem and its correlates, Shapiro et al. (1968) concluded that:

> During the 1940s maternal and child health programs at the state and local levels were greatly strengthened, and infant mortality was a prime target of health department activities. The Federal Emergency Maternity and Infant Care Program, designed to meet the urgent needs of wives and infants of men in the Armed Forces during World War II, helped bring regular prenatal and infant health supervision to broad segments of the population. This program ended after World War II. A large part of the reduction in infant loss was concentrated in the control of infectious diseases, whose toll was still substantial at the beginning of the 1940s. In some areas the introduction of special programs for the care of prematurely born infants also had an impact on the mortality rate. In the 1950s a general

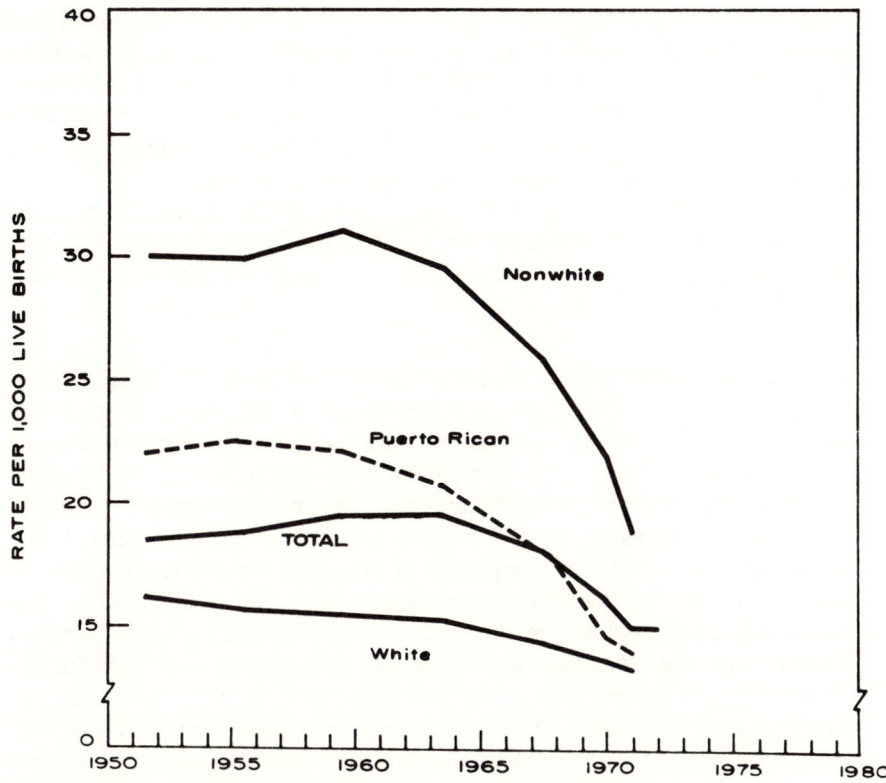

Figure 2. Neonatal Mortality Rates in New York City by Ethnic Group, 1950–71
Source: Pakter and Nelson 1974, 858.
Note: Rates for 1950–69 are four-year averages.

attitude that significant progress in reducing infant mortality required, above all, new insights into basic biological processes tended to dampen the fervor for action programs. The 1950s might also be characterized as a decade in which earlier medical and program advances in maternal and child health continued without significant innovations. This occurred in the absence of major scientific breakthroughs that could have been expected to produce broad effects through immediate application.

Finally, some of the very conditions which, on the surface, might be taken as harbingers of improvement had the reverse result. An outstanding example is the migration of nonwhite persons to large metropolitan areas; in many of these areas, infant mortality increased instead of decreasing. The explanation encompasses many social, economic, and program issues. High on the list would be a lag in community facilities in providing for the change, difficulties experienced by the in-migrant group in taking advantage of their new medical care environment, overcrowding, and low income. (pp. 136–37)

In contrast to the 15 years prior to 1965, an abrupt but continuing decline in NMR characterized the subsequent 15 years.

A survey of legitimate births conducted during 1964-66 concluded that approximately one fourth of all (not only neonatal) infant deaths were in excess of those expected on the basis of rates in the most favored socioeconomic class (Holtzman 1977). Kessner's results suggested that if all mothers had prenatal care equivalent to that provided to mothers with adequate care, the infant mortality rate would be 16 percent lower (Kessner 1973).

The abrupt and persistent decline since 1965 and the theoretical calculations indicating potential benefit from a reduction in the disparity between disadvantaged and other population groups suggested that medical care could influence the NMR.

In fact, there was evidence that medical care of particular types had an impact even during the relatively static decade of the 1950s. Shapiro and colleagues (1958, 1960) found that perinatal mortality (stillbirths plus early neonatal deaths) during 1955-57 was lower in a prepaid group practice (the Health Insurance Plan, or HIP) than elsewhere in New York City, even as compared with populations receiving care from private physicians. HIP's lower rates were not a consequence of selection for particular types of families defined by paternal occupation (a proxy for social class). It is possible that a higher percentage of deliveries attended by board-certified obstetricians (than was the case in the city as a whole) accounted for the effect, since there were major differences in mortality rates in the city between patients delivering on general service and those delivered by private physicians both for whites and nonwhites and regardless of occupational classification.

Shah and Abbey (1971), in a binary variable multiple regression analysis of births in Baltimore in 1960-64, showed that the effect of prenatal care on neonatal mortality varied but in all cases no care led to a worse outcome even after controlling for the sociodemographic variables of race, socioeconomic status, and maternal age.

Gortmacher's multivariate analysis (1979), using data on white legitimate births in the National Natality and Infant Mortality Survey, indicated that being born in a hospital attenuated the extent to which poverty was directly related to incidence of neonatal mortality rates. At least at that point in time, prior to implementation of the programs of the mid-1960s, there was evidence that neonatal intensive care units (NICUs) and other medical care programs facilitated the survival of high-risk infants who had access to such care. As there was no excess neonatal mortality among poor infants weighing under 2,500 grams, the excess (presumably among infants over 2,500 grams) was attributed to poorer care for infants not at obvious high risk due to low birth weight or prior pregnancy loss experienced by the mother.

A more recent demonstration of the impact of organizational factors on neonatal mortality was provided by a clinical trial in Madera County, California (Levy et al. 1971). In that study, delivery of prenatal care by nurse midwives resulted in significant reductions in the neonatal mortality rate in the county; subsequent reversion to care by physicians resulted in an increase in the neonatal mortality rate.

Even though prepaid group practice and care by nurse practitioners have become more common in the years since these studies were conducted, only a very small proportion of the population is exposed to such modes of organization. The remarkable decline in neonatal mortality must be attributable largely to other phenomena. Unfortunately, attribution of cause is difficult because of the existence of so many influences including the many sociodemographic characteristics (the most important of which are parity, maternal age, prior pregnancy experience, and social class) and the interactions among them (Harris 1982). Nevertheless, several studies provide evidence for the beneficial impact of medical care.

The Maternity and Infant Care Projects initiated in the mid-1960s had a relatively small impact on neonatal mortality rates. At least part of the lack of effect was a result of the relatively small proportion of the population served by these programs (Davis and Schoen 1978, 149). Despite this overall lack of impact, analyses of data from at least some of the local programs showed a reduction in neonatal mortality from rates of approximately 22 per 1,000 to about 15 per 1,000, that is, to a rate comparable to the nation as a whole in 1970 (152).

Davis and Reynolds (1976) found that Medicaid had only a slight effect on neonatal mortality rates once family planning and abortion were considered, and the effect was primarily in black populations.

Norris and Williams (1984) studied the impact of the California Medicaid program, introduced in 1966, on the perinatal death rate in the state in 1968 and 1978. The deaths examined were those occurring at 20 or more weeks' gestation through the first 27 days of life; thus fetal as well as neonatal mortality was considered. Standardized mortality rates were lower among Medicaid recipients, particularly in 1978, and especially when compared with non-Medicaid births occurring to women delivering in county hospitals, the population group most like the Medicaid group in sociodemographic characteristics.

The absence of data on a comparable population before the institution of the Medicaid program and the inability to control for the possible beneficial selection bias of relatively low-risk women into the Medicaid program were partially offset by the use of standardized mortality rates that were computed by adjusting crude mortality rates for age of mother, parity, birth weight, and race-ethnicity. Both the Medicaid and non-Medicaid groups increased their use of prenatal care between the two time periods, and both groups had the same frequency of four important procedures (fetal monitoring, amniocentesis, ultrasound, and Cesarean section), so the beneficial impact of Medicaid was not a result of increased exposure to these interventions. The study did not examine other factors (such as receipt of neonatal intensive care, family planning service, or the availability of abortions) that might have, at least partly, accounted for the effect.

Grossman and Jacobowitz's multivariate analysis (1981) of data from 1966–68 and 1970–72 demonstrated the predominant effect of legalized abortions on NMR. This study employed data on counties, obtained from the Area Resources File, the AMA (for physicians), and the American Hospital Association (for facilities). Only counties with populations of at least 50,000 and with at least 5,000 nonwhites were included in the study. The major variables were availability of Medicaid coverage for pregnancies (which varies from state to state), family planning facilities, maternity and infant care (M&I) facilities, and the legality of abortion (which varied by state). Control variables included maternal schooling, poverty characteristics of the county, race, and the physician-population ratio. The effect of legalized abortions was the most important factor in reducing both white and nonwhite neonatal mortality rates, an effect which dominated schooling and poverty and which was particularly pronounced among blacks. Prior to the legalization of abortion, which did not lead to an increase in abortions until the early 1970s, increased use of family planning clinics was the most important factor accounting for the decline in NMR between 1964 and 1971; after the legalization of abortion, family planning was the second most important factor. The third most important factor was Medicaid, which accounted for an additional 0.5 to 1.0 percent reduction in deaths per 1,000 live births. Maternal and infant care projects also had a small additional effect, especially on nonwhites. Grossman and Jacobowitz (1981) concluded:

> After a period of relative stability, neonatal mortality rates began to decline after 1964 as a lagged response to the extremely rapid increase in the percent of females who used the pill and the IUD between 1961 and 1964. The decline was further fueled by the increase in percent of low-income women who used subsidized family planning services between 1965 and 1971 and by a dramatic rise in the legal abortion rate between 1969 and 1971. An acceleration in the rate of decline in mortality rate between 1971 and 1977 was due primarily to the literal explosion of the abortion rate in that period. (p. 709)

In 1969, the U.S. rate of abortions was approximately 4 per 1,000. By 1982, it had risen to 400 per 1,000. Grossman and Jacobowitz estimated that a reimposed ban on abortions resulting in a return to the 1969 level would lead to an estimated increase in the NMR of 2.8 deaths per 1,000 nonwhite births and 1.8 deaths per 1,000 white births. If the use of other birth control methods did not compensate for the discontinued abortions, the increase in neonatal mortality would be 19 percent and 21 percent, respectively, above the 1977 levels.

Grossman and Jacobowitz (1981) also commented on certain studies which produced contradictory findings. In those studies, no controls for other determinants of infant mortality were employed, mortality was not race-specific, and the effect of abortion on neonatal mortality was not assessed.

Hadley's analysis (1982) of differences in neonatal mortality in 1969–73 between counties grouped according to economic criteria also provides evidence of the effect of medical care. Using the Area Resources File to characterize counties, he conducted a retrospective multivariate analysis, categorizing variables as those related to social policy (Medicaid coverage of pregnancy in its different forms, liberalization of abortion) and those related to medical care (number of abortions per 1,000 live births, number of obstetricians per 1,000 live births, proportion of physicians over 65 years old, proportion of physicians not board certified, proportion of hospitals with neonatal intensive care units, and Medicare expenditures per enrollee, which was used as a proxy for medical care expenditures overall). Maternal age and place of birth (in hospital or not) were included as sociodemographic variables. In this study, the effect of medical care was positive and similar across racial groups. Major findings were that an increase in medical care expenditures (as measured by Medicare expenditures per enrollee) decreased infant mortality by 1.5–2 percent, and an increase in physician/population ratio of 10 percent was associated with a decrease in infant mortality rate of 0.6–0.8 percent. The beneficial effect was considerably greater for postneonatal mortality than for neonatal mortality in blacks but only marginally so in whites. As was the case in the Grossman/Jacobowitz study (1981), the impact of legalized abortions was significant; the absolute reduction in neonatal mortality was greater for blacks although the rate of decline was greater for whites. The estimated impact of reductions in the abortion rate to its 1969 figure (4 per 1,000) would be to increase NMR by 25 percent for whites and 6 percent for blacks. The effect of Medicaid coverage of prenatal care also was to decrease NMR, especially among blacks; states whose Medicaid program did not cover unborn children had 2–5 percent higher NMR rates (or an equivalent of 28–107 excess deaths per 100,000 population).

In summary, several analyses of data using national samples and employing a large number of pertinent variables indicate that a variety of changes occurring since the mid-1960s have had a significant impact in reducing neonatal mortality. Of all the interventions, legalized abortion probably had the greatest effect. Family planning activities, which antedated the legalization of abortion, also had a major effect. Medicaid coverage of prenatal care was also related to improved pregnancy outcomes (decreased NMR).

However, despite Hadley's finding (1982) that the proportion of hospitals with NICUs was not associated with differences in neonatal mortality, an extensive literature documents the significant effect of improved technology in reducing infant mortality. In Hadley's study the proportion of hospitals with NICUs was used as a proxy for adequacy of neonatal intensive care; however, recent studies show that regionalization of services involving centralization of highly specialized facilities—the converse of what Hadley was measuring—is likely to be responsible for effective neonatal intensive care (see McCormick et al. 1984). In some areas of the country in which low birth weight ratios were initially high, declines in low birth weight accounted for as much as half of the decline in neonatal mortality in the late 1960s and early 1970s (David and Siegel 1983). However, several analyses have documented the fact that, for the country as a whole, the declines in neonatal mortality were largely birth weight-specific. Lee and colleagues (1980) conducted a retrospective ecological analysis of neonatal mortality and showed that declines in NMR since 1965 have been within each birth weight group. Since the decline in NMR was not a result of decreases in risk of mortality (as measured by low birth weight rates, which declined only slightly since 1968), it must have been a result of improvements in perinatal care, i.e., in events surrounding birth and neonatal care. Similar conclusions were reached by Williams and Chen (1982), Kleinman et al. (1978) and Harris (1982). Harris constructed and tested a continuous time stochastic model to study the effect of medical care on birth weight and neonatal mortality. In this study, which was restricted to births to black women in Massachusetts using data from 1975-76, Harris found only a weak relationship between prenatal care and birth weight-specific perinatal mortality and found that prenatal care was associated much more with increased gestation age and only slightly with increased birth weight. Harris concluded that the effect of prenatal care was to identify pregnancies at high risk and to facilitate access to effective perinatal care, at least in blacks. Moreover, in his study, the annual volume of deliveries in the hospital of birth had a significant effect on the survival of neonates.

In contrast to the lack of evidence of impact of prenatal care on low birth weight (see chap. 4), there is ample support for an effect of perinatal intensive care on neonatal mortality. Demographic shifts did not account for much of the decline in NMR in the study by Morris et al. (1975). They showed that only a small fraction of the observed improvement in birth weight-specific mortality represented favorable shifts in maternal age and poverty. On the other hand, advances in transport systems to regional centers, treatment of Rh-incompatibility, and treatment of respiratory distress syndrome could be expected to greatly facilitate care for the major causes of neonatal mortality (congenital anomalies, immaturity and related conditions, and relatively less severe instances of neonatal asphyxia).

A recent analysis using data from the major studies of the effectiveness of neonatal intensive care (Budetti and McManus 1982) provided conclusive evidence of the beneficial role of neonatal intensive care. Since 1970, 88 percent of the decline in infant mortality has been experienced in the neonatal period, even though only about 70 percent of the infant deaths were neonatal. Although only one randomized controlled clinical trial of neonatal intensive care has been conducted (Kitchen et al. 1978), its findings of benefit have been confirmed by epidemiologic surveys showing a relationship in time between the fall in NMR and organization of NICUs (Budetti and McManus 1982) and by reports from individual intensive care nurseries. Of the eight reports from individual units that presented birth weight-specific death rates, seven showed impressive declines over time. Budetti and McManus pooled data from studies of infants born in several hospitals into five-year periods beginning in 1961; the data demonstrate significant declines over time for infants with very low birth weight: declines from 50 percent to 20 percent in infants of birth weight 1,000–1,500 grams and from 93 percent to 50 percent in mortality of infants under 1,000 grams. Kitchen's study was able to demonstrate that staff experience and the nature of the newborn's problem rather than specific technology (such as continuous positive airway pressure) are critical factors in lowering the mortality in NICUs. Thus, although it is not possible to identify the precise intervention responsible for the effectiveness of NICUs or to determine whether NICUs can improve mortality without adopting the most advanced instrumentation (Hughes-Davies 1979), it is clear that they have had a salutary effect in reducing neonatal mortality.

Despite this evidence of effectiveness, however, the disparity in national neonatal mortality rates between poor and nonpoor infants failed to narrow. That is, the percentage of reduction in neonatal mortality was greater for the nonpoor than for the poor (Davis and Schoen 1978). This was also the case with regard to the decline in white versus nonwhite rates: white neonatal mortality declined 46 percent from 1965 to 1977, whereas nonwhite rates declined 42 percent (USDHEW 1980). Neonatal intensive care, in contrast to Medicaid, community health centers, and public family planning efforts, is not targeted specifically at any subgroup of the population defined by social characteristics. Although little is known about the financing of NICUs, only 17 percent of the total hospital charges for neonatal intensive care at Denver's Children's Hospital were charged to Medicaid in 1976, and only 12 percent of the charges were paid by Medicaid (McCarthy et al. 1979). At the Johns Hopkins Hospital, the comparable figure was only 40 percent (M Rogers, personal communication) even though about 40 percent of white births and 47 percent of nonwhite births in Baltimore are to socioeconomically deprived individuals as defined by less than a high school education (Strobino 1982) and the need for neonatal intensive care is much greater in these disadvantaged populations. Moreover, Medicaid coverage does not always extend to neonatal intensive care. In only three states is it clear that the state will pay for such care without special application for it (Davidson et al. 1982). States differ widely in the procedures required for verification of applicability, the extent to which they make coverage retroactive, and limitations on the duration of care.

Therefore, although NICUs have undoubtedly been responsible for much of the decline in neonatal mortality in the period from 1965 to 1979, only programs that are uniquely suited to meet the needs of the poor (such as easier access to abortions, family planning, and special programs for prenatal care) have been effective in reducing some of the excess of neonatal mortality among the poor where the programs are well developed.

References

Budetti P, McManus P. Assessing the effectiveness of neonatal intensive care. Med Care 1982;20:1027-39.

David R, Siegel E. Declines in neonatal mortality, 1968 and 1977: better babies or better care? Pediatrics 1983;71:531-40.

Davidson S, Simon M, Connelly J. Interstate variation in Medicaid coverage of newborns. Report of phase I. Working paper no. 8. Department of Health Systems Research and Development. American Academy of Pediatrics. Elk Grove Village, Ill., May 1982.

Davis K, Reynolds R. The impact of Medicare and Medicaid on access to medical care. In: Rosett R, ed. The role of health insurance in the health services sector. New York: Neale Watson Academic Publications for the National Bureau of Economic Research, 1976:391-425.

Davis K, Schoen C. Health and the war on poverty: a ten-year appraisal. Washington, D.C.: Brookings Institution, 1978.

Glass L, Evans H, Swartz D, Rajegowda B, Leblanc W. Effects of legalized abortion on neonatal mortality and obstetrical morbidity at Harlem Hospital Center. Am J Public Health 1974;64:717-78.

Gortmacher S. Poverty and infant mortality in the United States. Am Sociol Rev 1979;44:280-97.

Grossman M, Jacobowitz S. Variations in infant mortality rates among counties of the United States: the roles of public policies and programs. Demography 1981;18:695-713.

Hadley J. More medical care, better health? Washington, D.C.: Urban Institute Press, 1982.

Harris J. Prenatal medical care and infant mortality. In: Fuchs V, ed. Economic aspects of health. Chicago: University of Chicago Press, 1982:15-52.

Holtzman N. The goal of preventing early death. In: Blendon R, Duval M, Hiscock W, eds. Conditions for change in the health system. USDHEW public health service. Washington, D.C.: U.S. Government Printing Office, 1977:107-32. (DHEW publication no. (HRA) 78-642).

Hughes-Davies T. Conservative care of the newborn baby. Arch Dis Child 1979;54:59-61.

Kessner D. Infant death: an analysis by maternal risk and health care. Washington, D.C.: Institute of Medicine, National Academy of Sciences, 1973.

Kitchen W, Ryan M, Rickards A. A longitudinal study of very low-birthweight infants. Dev Med Child Neurol 1978;20:605-18.

Kleinman J, Kovar M, Feldman J, Young C. A comparison of 1960 and 1973-1974 early neonatal mortality in selected states. Am J Epidemiol 1978;108:454-69.

Lanman J, Kohl S, Bedell J. Changes in pregnancy outcome after liberalization of the New York State abortion law. Am J Obstet Gynecol 1974;118:485-92.

Lee S, Paneth N, Gartner L, Pearlman M, Gross L. Neonatal mortality: an analysis of the recent improvement in the United States. Am J Public Health 1980;70:15-21.

Levy B, Wilkinson F, Marine W. Reducing neonatal mortality rate with nurse-midwives. Am J Obstet Gynecol 1971;109:50-58.

McCarthy J, Koops B, Honeyfield P, Butterfield LJ. Who pays the bill for neonatal intensive care? J Pediatr 1979;95:755-62.

McCormick M, Shapiro S, Starfield B. The regionalization of perinatal services: summary of the evaluation of a national demonstration program. JAMA 1984; 253:799-804.

Morris N, Udry J, Chase C. Shifting age-parity distribution of births and the decrease in infant mortality. Am J Public Health 1975;65:359-62.

Norris F, Williams R. Perinatal outcomes among Medicaid recipients in California. Am J Public Health 1984;74:1112-17.

Pakter J, Nelson F. Factors in the unprecedented decline in infant mortality in New York City. Bull NY Acad Med 1974;50:839-68.

Shah F, Abbey H. Effects of some factors on neonatal and postneonatal mortality. Milbank Mem Fund Q 1971;49:33-57.

Shapiro S, Jacobziner H, Densen P, Weiner L. Further observations on prematurity and perinatal mortality in a general population and in the population of a prepaid group practice medical care plan. Am J Public Health 1960;50:1304-17.

Shapiro S, Schlesinger E, Nesbitt R. Infant, perinatal, maternal, and childhood mortality in the United States. Cambridge, Mass.: Harvard University Press, 1968.

Shapiro S, Weiner L, Densen P. Comparison of prematurity and perinatal mortality in a general population and in the population of a prepaid group practice medical care plan. Am J Public Health 1958;48:170-87.

Strobino D. Trends in low birth weight infants and changes in Baltimore's childbearing population, 1972-77. Public Health Rep 1982;97:273-82.

USDHEW. Health of the disadvantaged. Chart Book-II, 1980:38 (DHEW publication no. (HRA)80-633).

Williams R, Chen P. Identifying the sources of the recent decline in perinatal mortality rates in California. N Engl J. Med 1982;306:207-14.

3
Postneonatal Mortality

Barbara Starfield

Mortality rates in the first year of life have declined markedly since the turn of the century. This decline is due largely to great reductions in postneonatal mortality—that is, deaths during the second through eleventh months of life (Pharoah and Morris 1979). In contrast to the situation with neonatal mortality (death during the first 27 days of life), where the impact of technologic and organizational changes are evident, changes in postneonatal mortality have historically been influenced primarily by changing social conditions, at least up to the mid-1960s. Figure 3 shows that from 1915 to 1930, when there were major improvements in nutrition and sanitation, the decline in postneonatal mortality was relatively greater than the decline in neonatal mortality. In the 1930s, the implementation of legislation to increase access to medical care was associated with an accelerated decline in neonatal mortality and a continued decline in postneonatal mortality. These declines persisted into the 1940s coincident with the federal Emergency Maternity and Infant Care Program designed to meet the urgent needs of wives and infants of servicemen in World War II. This program ended after the war and the rate of decline in postneonatal mortality slowed in the 1950s; by 1960 the rate of decline in neonatal mortality was extremely small and postneonatal mortality did not decline at all.

Reasons for declines in postneonatal mortality prior to 1965 are relatively clear (Shapiro et al. 1968, 124). Higher rates of mortality from infectious disease of the digestive and respiratory tract and from accidents accounted for almost the entire gap between postneonatal mortality rates (PNMR) in the United States and other industrialized countries at a time when the United States ranked close to the highest among the low infant mortality countries (Shapiro et al. 1968; Pharoah and Morris 1979). The leveling off of the decline in postneonatal mortality resulting from influenza and pneumonia that started in the 1950s was not paralleled in these other countries except in England and Wales, which showed trends similar to those in the United States. Moreover, the postneonatal death rate for respiratory illnesses other

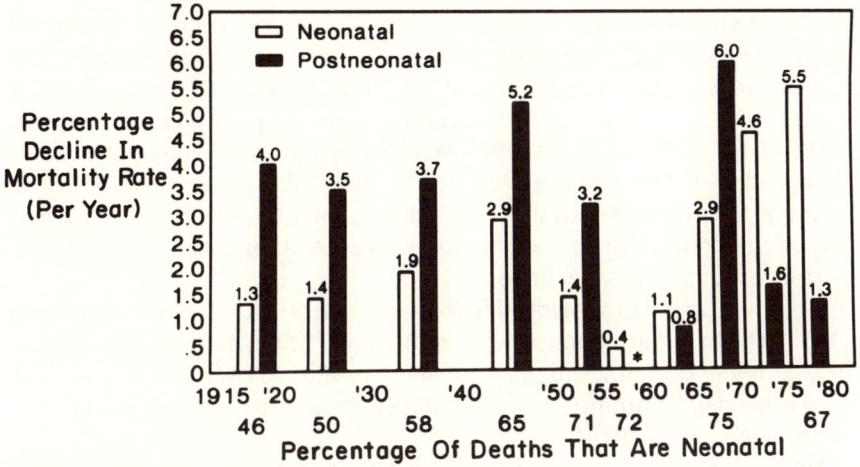

Figure 3. Percentage Decline in Infant Mortality, 1915–80
Source: Starfield 1984.
*Percentage decline in postneonatal mortality rate was 0.0 from 1955 to 1960.

than influenza and pneumonia rose throughout the 1950s and into the early 1960s, whereas it declined elsewhere (except England and Wales). In comparison with those in the United States, deaths associated with congenital anomalies accounted for a larger proportion of postneonatal deaths in these countries, although the actual PNMR from congenital anomalies was similar (Shapiro et al. 1968).

The potential but unrealized impact of medical care on PNMR in the pre-1965 period was demonstrated by Gortmacher (1979) in a study of white legitimate births. In contrast to the situation with neonatal mortality, where poor infants identified as high-risk did as well as nonpoor infants at high risk, no such attenuating effect was found in the case of PNMR. That is, poor infants of low birth weight or with older siblings did worse than nonpoor infants of low birth weight or with older siblings with regard to their likelihood of survival to one year of age. The finding led Gortmacher to conclude that whereas well-developed tertiary care centers were able to overcome the adverse effects of poverty in the neonatal period and in infants who gained entrance into the system, the ability of the system to identify and deal with health needs was compromised in the case of poor infants once they left the hospital for the community.

Figure 3 shows that an abrupt and large decline in postneonatal mortality occurred after 1965, coincident with legislation associated with the War on Poverty, and in the late 1960s the decline was greater than at any time since the 1940s. Since 1970, the rate of decline has slowed markedly and in 1977–79 there was no decrease at all in the country as a whole (Starfield 1985).

A feature of the decline in postneonatal mortality during the 1965–79 period was a narrowing of the gap between whites and nonwhites (Davis and Schoen 1978, 32). Nearly all of the improvement in the infant mortality rate of nonwhites relative to whites occurred in the postneonatal period. Equally notable was the narrowing of the gap between the poor and the nonpoor, although the evidence is indirect. Davis and Schoen (34) arrayed the states into groups of ten characterized by the proportion of families living in poverty. Between 1965 and 1979 infant mortality rates declined more rapidly in the poorer states, and the poorer the group of states, the more the postneonatal mortality declined.

Goldman and Grossman's lagged-time series multivariate regression (1978) showed that counties with community health centers experienced greater relative declines in postneonatal mortality between 1970 and 1978 than in neonatal mortality. These counties also experienced reductions in the white/nonwhite disparity.

Hadley's analysis (1982) of 1969–73 data from counties arrayed according to economic criteria into over 400 county groups indicated the positive effect of higher medical expenditures (as measured by the proxy variable Medicare expenditures per Medicare enrollee) and more pediatricians per 1,000 live births. (Unfortunately, his analysis of correlates of postneonatal mortality did not include any variables comparable to Medicaid coverage, as was possible in the neonatal analyses.) In these analyses, differences in birth weight distributions in the county groups were controlled by the incorporation of a variable applying 1960 birth weight–specific mortalities to these distributions. The magnitude of the effect of medical expenditures and pediatricians was greater for blacks than for whites although all effects in both males and females were statistically significant at the 99 percent confidence level. It is noteworthy that the effect of the medical care variables was about five times greater for postneonatal mortality than it was for neonatal mortality in black infants; for white infants the effect was only marginally greater for postneonatal mortality.

Disparities between the poor and nonpoor are greatest in the postneonatal period (Pharoah and Morris 1979; Antonovsky and Bernstein 1977). Although much of this disparity is a result of other sociodemographic factors associated with social class (such as poverty, education, and maternal age) (MacMahon et al. 1970), the fact that it can be reduced in the absence of major changes in sociodemographic factors and coincident with increases in the provision of medical services suggests that medical care can and almost certainly does have a significant impact. In an inquiry into the causes of 187 postneonatal deaths in England and Wales it was found that 23 percent of the avoidable factors were attributable to medical services and 71 percent were social or parental in origin, including failure to seek care. In a subsequent study of 226 deaths in Glasgow, half of all deaths occurred at home, and many of the children admitted to the hospital were already critically ill. In New Zealand, only 20 percent of infants were in the hospital at the time of death. Pharoah and Morris (1979) interpret the data from these and other studies to indicate that families from the lower social classes do not seek care in proportion to their needs, but the extent to which this can be overcome by better medical care services is not addressed.

The study conducted by Bradshaw et al. (1982) provides evidence on this point. After controlling for level of unemployment, the proportion of larger families (a variable related to poverty), the proportion of lone-parent families, and level of overcrowding, the variation between areas in rates of infant mortality persisted, leading the authors to conclude that differences in health and social services were responsible for at least some of the variation. (They recognized that not all relevant sociodemographic factors were incorporated into their regression equations.) Unfortunately, the study did not separate neonatal from postneonatal mortality so that it is impossible to determine the nature of the impact.

Thus although the effect of medical care specifically on postneonatal mortality has been relatively poorly studied, evidence supports the conclusion that postneonatal mortality is responsive to changes in the provision of medical care such as those that occurred during certain periods in the recent past.

References

Antonovsky A, Bernstein J. Social class and infant mortality. Soc Sci Med 1977;11:453–70.

Bradshaw J, Edwards H, Lawton D, Staden F, Weale J, Weekes A. Variations in infant mortality 1975–1977. J Epidemiol Community Health 1982;36:11–16.

Davis K, Schoen C. Health and the war on poverty: A ten-year appraisal. Washington, D.C.: Brookings Institution, 1978.

Goldman F, Grossman M. The impact of public health policy: the case of community health centers. Cambridge, Mass: National Bureau of Economic Research, 1978, working paper no. 1020.

Gortmacher S. Poverty and infant mortality in the United States. Am Sociol Rev 1979;44:280–97.

Hadley J. More medical care, better health? Washington, D.C.: Urban Institute Press, 1982.

MacMahon B, Kovar M, Feldman J. Infant mortality rates: socioeconomic factors. USDHEW Vital Health Statistics, series 22, no. 14, 1970.

Pharoah P, Morris J. Postneonatal mortality. Epidemiol Rev 1979;1:170–83.

Shapiro S, Schlesinger E, Nesbitt R. Infant, perinatal, maternal, and childhood mortality in the United States. Cambridge, Mass.: Harvard University Press, 1968.

Starfield B. Social factors in childhood illness. In: Green M, Haggerty R. Ambulatory pediatrics III. Philadelphia: W. B. Saunders Co., 1984:13.

Starfield B. Postneonatal mortality. Ann Rev Public Health. 1985;6:21–40.

4
Low Birth Weight

Barbara Starfield

Low birth weight (LBW) is a major determinant of adverse outcome of pregnancy. It is associated with about 75 percent of neonatal deaths and 30 percent of postneonatal deaths, even though the frequency of LBW is only on the order of 6–7 percent. For infants weighing 2,500 grams or less at birth, the neonatal death rate is almost 40 times as great as it is for infants weighing over 2,500 grams; infants 2,500 grams or less at birth are five times as likely to die in the postneonatal period (Shapiro et al. 1980).

LBW can be attributed to a variety of factors. The relative importance of these factors as contributors to the problem was examined in a review of existing literature that categorized them as related to maternal diseases (those related and those not related to pregnancy), placental disease, infant factors (such as multiple births or congenital defects), and social factors (including smoking, poor nutrition, and poor physical condition) (Hemminki and Starfield 1978). The most important factors appeared to be those related to poor nutrition and poor physical condition. Although poverty has generally been considered a major correlate of LBW (NCHS 1972a), Gortmacher (1979b) demonstrated that poverty had no direct effect on LBW when other sociodemographic variables were included in the analysis, at least in this study of white legitimate births in 1964–65. This finding confirms the suspicion that poverty affects birth weight largely through its effect on factors such as nutrition and physical condition. Analyses from the 1972 national survey show that the higher frequency of LBW among the poor occurs at or near term (Placek 1977). As the proportion of infants who are premature (born at less than 37 weeks of gestation) is only slightly higher for poor infants, the excess of LBW is primarily due to a greater likelihood of intrauterine growth retardation. Therefore, medical care will be effective in reducing the disparity in LBW rates between the poor and the nonpoor primarily to the extent that it has an impact on factors associated with intrauterine growth; an effect that is primarily associated with prolongation of gestation alone is not likely to have much impact with regard to reducing disparities between the poor and nonpoor.

Trends in LBW, 1950–64

In the United States as a whole, LBW ratios increased during the 15-year period 1950 to 1964 (Table 1), from 7.5 in 1950 to 7.7 in 1960 to 8.2 in 1964 (NCHS 1980a). The increase was limited to nonwhite births: in 1950 the ratio was 10.2 and it increased to 12.8 in 1960 and 13.9 in 1964 whereas the comparable data for whites were 7.1, 6.8, and 7.1. The increase was noted in all birth weight groups of 2,500 grams or less, but proportionally the increase was greater in lower birth weight groups (NCHS 1972b; Shapiro et al. 1968, 317). The increase in LBW infants among nonwhites occurred in the absence of an increase in the proportion of births that were premature (less than 37 weeks gestation) (NCHS 1972b, 9–10); if the increase in LBW had been due only to in-migrations of at-risk populations or better registration of births, a change in distribution of gestation age would have been expected. The increase was also not attributable to changing distributions of live births by age of mother, plurality, or sex. Unfortunately, national data for the period 1950–64 do not provide information on the relationship between socioeconomic characteristics and birth weight, so it is possible that the increase in proportions of LBW among nonwhite births was associated with socioeconomic factors during that period (NCHS 1972b). Shapiro et al. suggest that it is possible that the increase was due to better registration of births and/or demographic migrations into areas with better reporting of births but indicate that the increase was "too general, occurring in almost every type of geographic area, to be primarily accounted for in this way" (1968, 50).

Trends in LBW, 1965–79

The percentage of infants with birth weight of 2,500 grams or less reached a peak in 1965–66 and declined progressively thereafter. Table 2 indicates that this decline has been evident for both white and nonwhite births and in urban as well as nonurban areas, although the decline for nonwhite births in nonurban areas was delayed for an additional three years (until 1968–69) (Chase 1977).

The marked change in LBW in the mid-1960s is strikingly shown in Figure 4, which contains data from New York City. After rising for a decade, the proportion of infants who were of LBW fell after 1965 in both races but particularly among nonwhites (Pakter and Nelson 1974).

The effect of medical care in reducing the occurrence of LBW is a subject of considerable controversy. Although there is much that can be done to reduce the poor prognosis associated with serious conditions such as diabetes in pregnancy, vaginal bleeding, and hypertension, the benefit to be expected from routine prenatal care is difficult to specify. There is no single intervention that is targeted at the prevention of LBW, and there is considerable potential for harm from the application of sophisticated technology (includ-

Table 1
Percentage of Infants Weighing 2,500 Grams or Less at Birth, United States, 1950–64

	All Births	White	Nonwhite
1950	7.5	7.1	10.2
1951	7.5	7.0	10.7
1952	7.6	7.0	11.1
1953	7.6	7.0	11.3
1954	7.4	6.8	11.3
1955	7.6	6.8	11.7
1956	7.5	6.7	12.0
1957	7.6	6.8	12.4
1958	7.7	6.8	12.9
1959	7.7	6.8	12.9
1960	7.7	6.8	12.8
1961	7.8	6.9	13.0
1962	8.0	7.0	13.1
1963	8.2	7.1	13.6
1964	8.2	7.1	13.9

Source: NCHS 1980a, 24.

ing routine screening) in otherwise uncomplicated pregnancies (Enkin and Chalmers 1982). Although it is possible that certain aspects of prenatal care are particularly effective in preventing certain adverse effects, there is no compelling theoretical reason why routine prenatal care should reduce the likelihood of occurrence of LBW. Neither nutritional advice nor advice to stop smoking appear to be effective in reducing the frequency of LBW associated with poor nutrition or smoking, even when better nutritional practices are adopted or when the amount of smoking is decreased (Enkin and Chalmers 1982). It is perhaps this lack of a clear rationale that relates specific aspects of care to specific benefits that at least in part accounts for the inability of studies to consistently demonstrate that the amount of prenatal care influences the frequency of LBW.

A study conducted in 1968 concerning the experience in New York City indicated that among women who were at sociodemographic risk (based on age, education, birth order, and illegitimacy), the frequency of LBW among those who received inadequate prenatal care (four or fewer prenatal visits or none before the third trimester) was double that among those who received adequate care (Kessner 1973). Among women at neither sociodemographic nor medical-obstetric risk, those who received no care had LBW frequencies almost double (1.8 times higher) those receiving adequate care (Kessner 1973). Similar findings were reported by Shah and Abbey (1971). Following the introduction of nurse-midwives in Madera County, California, in 1960, the number of women receiving prenatal care and the number of visits per woman increased and the LBW rate decreased; termination of the program in 1963 led to an increase in the LBW frequency (Levy et al. 1971).

The Maternity and Infant Care (MIC) Projects succeeded in increasing the

Table 2
Percentage of Infants Weighing 2,500 Grams or Less at Birth, United States, 1965-79

	All Births	White	Nonwhite	Black	Urban Areas	Other Areas
1965	8.3	7.2	13.8	—	8.9	7.5
1966	8.3	7.2	13.9	—	9.0	7.5
1967	8.2	7.1	13.6	—	8.9	7.4
1968	8.2	7.1	13.7	—	8.8	7.5
1969	8.1	7.0	13.5	14.1	8.8	7.3
1970	7.9	6.8	13.3	13.9	8.5	7.2
1971	7.7	6.6	12.7	13.4	8.2	6.9
1972	7.7	6.5	12.9	13.6	8.3	6.9
1973	7.6	6.4	12.5	13.3	8.1	6.9
1974	7.4	6.3	12.4	13.1	8.0	6.7
1975	7.4	6.3	12.2	13.0	—	—
1976	7.3	6.1	12.1	13.0	—	—
1977	7.1	5.9	—	12.8	—	—
1978	7.1	5.9	11.9	12.9	—	—
1979	6.9	5.8	11.6	12.6	—	—
1980	6.8	5.7	11.5	12.5	—	—

Sources: Chase 1977, 22; NCHS 1979; NCHS 1980a, 24; NCHS 1980b; NCHS 1981; NCHS 1982; NCHS 1983, 123.

proportion of women entering care in the first trimester (with a doubling of the percentage between 1967 and 1972) and in reducing the proportion receiving care for the first time in the third trimester (from 10 to 5 percent between 1967 and 1972) (Maternal & Child Health Services 1973). However, these projects were not very successful in reducing the LBW ratio, which averaged 133 per 1,000 (as compared with 151 per 1,000 for black families in poverty areas and 93 per 1,000 for whites in poverty areas). Davis (1977) indicated that less than 13 percent of all births were represented in these programs, and these included substantial numbers of nonpoor families (226). Calculations by Davis and Schoen (1978) suggested that an LBW ratio of 114 per 1,000 would have been expected for the M&I areas (given that 62 percent of the population served was black). A national evaluation of these projects concluded that the outcomes of pregnancies among women enrolled was better than those in comparable women not enrolled in the areas in which the projects existed, although the differences in LBW ratio were not statistically significant (Tayback et al. 1973). Moreover, within individual projects, there was a significant inverse correlation between availability of nutritional advice and occurrence of LBW (Tayback et al. 1973). Other studies have shown that nutritional supplements reduce the likelihood of LBW (Pritchard and Whalley 1974), although nutritional supplementation among black women in a large prospective study in New York City failed to increase birth weight (Rush et al. 1980). Several studies of caloric supplementation in developing countries have shown beneficial effects including increased birth weight (Kennedy et al. 1982), but the authors of an extensive

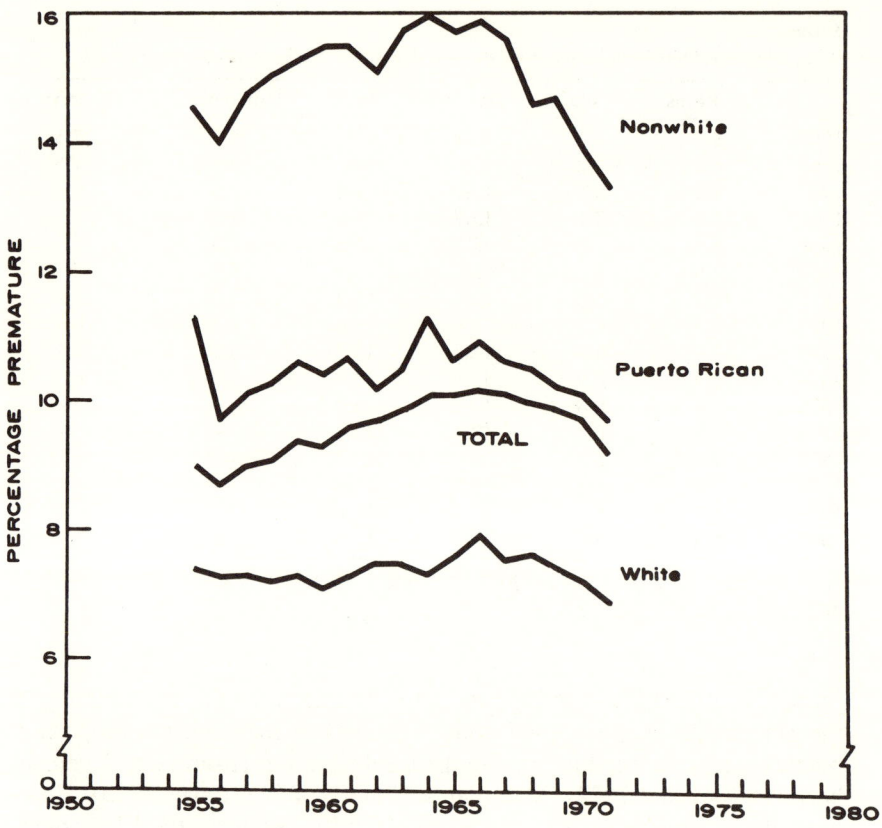

Figure 4. Incidence of Prematurity* in New York City by Ethnic Group, 1955–71
Source: Pakter and Nelson 1974, 850.
*Births of less than 2,501 grams

review of the evidence provided by controlled clinical trials published in the English, German, Finnish, and Scandinavian language concluded that there was no evidence to suggest benefit from the well-accepted routine administration of iron or vitamins in pregnancy (Hemminki and Starfield 1978).

Evaluations of the benefit of the Special Supplemental Food Program for Women, Infants, and Children (WIC) fail to provide conclusive evidence of the effectiveness of nutrition programs during pregnancy, but there have been few studies that were well designed and controlled. Three studies suggest that the program has some benefit. Data collected by Edozien et al. (1979) in an uncontrolled study of 19 primarily urban projects in 14 states provided evidence of a variety of benefits including that on birth weight. Although supplementation for a period less than three months had no effect on birth weight, supplementation of longer duration increased mean birth weight, even after controlling for an increase in gestational age. Unfortunately, the "follow-up" rate was only about 50 percent in the study with no information about the characteristics of women who did not return for follow-up. Also, the mean increase in birth weight was small and no distributions of birth weight were provided in the report. Kennedy et al. (1982) analyzed data on birth weight of infants born to Massachusetts women. This controlled trial studied the experiences of three categories of women: those in a WIC program; those who applied for a WIC program but could not participate because there were no openings or because they applied postpartum; and those cared for in non-WIC facilities. The women in these three groups were similar with regard to age, economic status, prior pregnancy outcome, weight, income, family size, number of living children, and obstetrical risk score. Birth weights were significantly higher among the WIC participants (mean 7.19 pounds, as compared with 6.92 pounds for the other groups combined and 6.88 for the first control group). The effect of a variety of other variables was also examined; among these, only prior pregnancy experience, gestational age, maternal weight gain, and smoking (but not income, prenatal care, or nutrition counseling within this generally low-income population) had a significant impact on birth weight. When these four variables were entered into a multiple regression with WIC participation, WIC remained a significant impact on birth weight. The well-known (though often not well-considered) confounding effect imposed by the fact that pregnancies destined to be longer provide a longer potential exposure for interventions was dealt with by the authors in a subanalysis, with persistence of an effect of WIC participation. No data on distributions of birth weight (for example, proportion under 2,500 grams) were provided. The third study demonstrating benefit from WIC participation (Hicks et al. 1982) compared 21 sibling pairs, one of whom had intrauterine exposure to WIC and the other of whom had exposure postnatally only. Those exposed prenatally performed better on a variety of cognitive and behavioral measures, but the small and not statistically significant effect on mean birth weight could be explained by the effect of greater parity among the early supplemented siblings.

An assessment of evidence from unpublished as well as published studies led the General Accounting Office (USGAO 1984) to conclude that on average there was a small but positive effect (1–2 percent) of WIC participation on mean birth weight and an approximate 16–20 percent decrease in the proportion of LBW infants. Although there were fewer data, those available suggested that WIC participation was particularly beneficial for women at highest risk.

Therefore, although evidence of benefit from programs to improve prenatal nutrition is mixed, there is some indication that certain interventions in particular population subgroups increase birth weight. It has been suggested that mean monthly weight gain during pregnancy could be used to determine which communities would benefit most from prenatal supplementation (Prentice et al. 1983).

Legalization of abortion also appears to have reduced the frequency of births of infants who are very small. Both Glass et al. (1974) and Lanman et al. (1974) showed a sharp decline in the incidence of birth weight under 1,000 grams after abortion was legalized.

A critical question is whether or not standard prenatal care has a significant impact on the occurrence of LBW. In 1969, 43 percent of black and 72 percent of white expectant mothers began prenatal care during their first trimester of pregnancy. By 1977, 59 percent and 77 percent, respectively, did so, and only 3 percent of expectant black mothers and 1 percent of expectant white mothers had no prenatal care (NCHS 1978, table A; Harris 1982, table 20).

Prenatal care is widely regarded as effective. In a classic and often cited study, Kessner (1973) showed a positive relationship between receipt of prenatal care and birth weight, using data from New York City in 1968. This study as well as the earlier Baltimore study reported by Shah and Abbey (1971), suggested that the impact of prenatal care may have resulted from its relationship with other factors rather than through its own effect. Moreover, the analyses were ecological so that it was not possible to determine whether the improvement in LBW in individuals was associated with receipt of prenatal care by those individuals.

Gortmacher (1979a) reanalyzed the New York City data using multidimensional contingency tables. Among both whites and blacks, except for white mothers delivering on private services, there was a substantially increased risk of LBW if prenatal care was inadequate (as opposed to adequate). The author was not able to rule out the possibility that the effects were due to selection of women with certain characteristics into prenatal care.

Greenberg (1983) analyzed birth certificates for U.S. births in 1977 and found that women who received no prenatal care were three times more likely to deliver an infant weighing less than 2,500 grams than women receiving some prenatal care. Although the relative risk of LBW with no prenatal care was greatest among white, highly educated women, the overall beneficial impact of prenatal care was greatest among the black, poorly educated population, because of the much greater frequency of both LBW and absence of prenatal care. As was the case with other studies using birth certificates, the unavailability of information on certain important correlates of LBW made it impossible to determine whether the observed effect of prenatal care was primary or a result of its association with some other more proximate factor.

Lewit (1983), using an econometric model, estimated the effect of prenatal service on LBW in New York City in the first six months of 1970. In this study, health districts were characterized according to the availability of M&I clinics, hours of clinic availability (both hospital and M&I), and number of obstetrician/gynecologists. Characteristics of prenatal care were time of the first visit and number of prenatal visits. Control variables included maternal and paternal education, prior pregnancy outcome, wantedness, legitimacy, and race. The greater the number of clinic hours available the greater the likelihood that prenatal care was sought at all but neither the presence of M&I clinics nor the number of obstetrician/gynecologists had an impact; the availability of clinic hours was greatest where paternal education (which was used as a proxy for income) was low. If prenatal care was received, paternal education was highly associated with the early seeking of care but the availability of resources did not appear to facilitate the early seeking of care. Only the number of clinic hours was related to the total number of prenatal visits, and only slightly so. Holding gestation age constant, there was a gain of 110 grams for each trimester care was sought earlier and the adverse effects of race and illegitimacy were reduced by an increasing number of visits, decreased interval to first visit, and receipt of any prenatal care.

Harris' analysis (1982) of black births in Massachusetts in 1975–76 employed a continuous time stochastic model to estimate the effect of prenatal care. The contribution of this study was its careful description and analysis of the complicated relationship between the timing of prenatal visits and the duration of pregnancy (and birth weight). Whereas most investigators have assumed a linear relationship between the number of visits and the length of gestation, Harris showed that this is not the case. His data indicated that prenatal care is associated with a decrease in preterm (under 36 weeks) delivery, even when the type of care (private or ward), percent in rented housing, median income of census tract, maternal education, and maternal age were controlled. However, women who receive care very early (in the first month) have higher rates of delivery under 36 weeks than women receiving care in the second or third months, which he attributed to perception of greater risk among these women. Prenatal care was found to have a greater effect on increasing gestational age than on increasing birth weight.

Thus, there is little firm evidence that the amount of prenatal care or even its timing by themselves have a substantial impact on birth weight.

Despite this conclusion, it appears that care of certain types (such as was provided in the controlled trial of Levy et al. 1971, mentioned above) can reduce the frequency of LBW rate in populations exposed to them.

One analysis of the impact of comprehensive (as compared with standard) prenatal care as provided by an MIC Project concluded that services such as more education, nutrition counseling, social services, and dental care were associated with better birth weight distributions (Sokol et al. 1980). Although it is possible that the beneficial effect was at least in part a result of the self-selection of women at lower risk into the institutions in which the study was conducted, an attempt was made to control for the major risk factors in the analysis of differences between women cared for in the MIC prenatal program and those receiving standard prenatal care. Of particular interest was the finding that the beneficial impact of comprehensive care on LBW appeared to be a result of improvements in intrauterine growth rather than prolongation of gestation, as the women enrolled in WIC were at higher risk of poor fetal growth but not at higher risk of premature labor. Therefore, it may be that approaches focusing specifically on risks such as smoking are responsible for the improvements. However, improvements in distribution of birth weight resulting from reductions in smoking will not necessarily reduce neonatal mortality rates (Rantakallio 1979) although they can be expected to result in better health of the offspring.

In a multivariate analysis of the relationship between the amount of prenatal care and birth weight among California births in 1978, Showstack et al. (1984) considered the number and timing of prenatal visits; their measure took into account the duration of gestation in calculating the number of visits considered to be "adequate" care. Adequate prenatal care was associated with increased birth weight, especially among black infants. Approximately one-half the improvement in birth weight was a result of increased duration of pregnancy whereas the other half was a direct effect on birth weight. Births in Kaiser hospitals, i.e., hospitals that are part of prepaid group practices, were related to both greater degrees of adequate prenatal care and higher mean birth weights.

Another analysis of the impact of prenatal care as provided by the Maternity and Infant Care Project was conducted by Peoples and Siegel (1983) in North Carolina. In this study, birth weights of infants born in counties served by the MIC Project were compared with birth weights of infants born in comparison counties selected on the basis of their similarities to the MIC counties with regard to socioeconomic status, health resources, and prior prenatal characteristics. Only births to mothers who made at least one prenatal visit were included. Although the availability of MIC services improved the extent to which prenatal care was considered adequate, there was no overall effect on the proportion of births that were of low birth weight. However, the population group at highest risk did appear to benefit from MIC services. Nonwhite teenagers in the MIC counties who were judged to have received adequate care (as determined by the number and pattern of visits) were less likely to have LBW infants than the nonwhite teenagers receiving adequate care in the comparison counties. The findings of this study add to the evidence that it is the content rather than the amount of care that is influential in reducing LBW in populations at high risk.

The experience of other large prepaid group practices is instructive in this regard. In the studies done in the 1950s in the Health Insurance Plan (HIP) of New York, LBW ratios were lower in births to patients in the plan than among other births in New York City regardless of the trimester in which care was sought, and within groups varying in prior pregnancy outcomes in both whites and blacks. When the HIP experience was compared only with that of patients seeing private physicians, the group practice patients had a lower frequency of LBW. More recent experience confirms the finding of a small advantage to HMO patients with regard to birth weight, despite a greater lag in starting prenatal care and a smaller number of visits in the HMO (Quick et al. 1982). In these organizations (HMOs and prepaid group practices), prenatal care is but one component in the ongoing care of the women enrolled. As Shapiro indicated, "the content of care may override the effect of a small difference in timing and frequency of prenatal care . . . we will not fully understand the potential of prenatal care in reducing the risk of low birth weight unless we jointly consider the timing, frequency, and content of care" (1981, 366).

As currently conceived, routine prenatal care and research related to the impact of components of prenatal care are not systematically addressed at understanding and dealing with the precise mechanisms accounting for the striking social class gradient in LBW (Enkin and Chalmers 1982). As it is possible that the determinants of LBW antedate pregnancy, the benefits of prenatal care may be realized only when they are part of a longer-term program of adequate health care, at least for populations at high risk.

References

Chase H. Time trends in low birth weight in the United States 1950–1974. In: Reed D, Stanley F, eds. The epidemiology of prematurity. Baltimore: Urban & Schwarzenberg, 1977:17–37.

Davis K. A decade of policy developments in providing health care for low-income families. In: Haveman R, ed. A decade of federal antipoverty programs. New York: Academic Press, 1977:197–231.

Davis K, Schoen C. Health and the war on poverty: a ten-year appraisal. Washington, D.C.: Brookings Institution, 1978.

Edozien J, Switzer B, Bryan R. Medical evaluation of the special supplemental food program for women, infants, and children. Am J Clin Nutr 1979;32:677–692.

Enkin M, Chalmers I. Effectiveness and satisfaction in antenatal care. In: Enkin M, Chalmers I, eds. Effectiveness and satisfaction in Antenatal Care. Philadelphia: Lippincott, 1982:266–290.

Glass L, Evans H, Swartz D, Rajegowda B, Leblanc W. Effects of legalized abortion on neonatal mortality and obstetrical morbidity at Harlem Hospital Center. Am J Public Health 1974;64:717–18.

Gortmacher S. The effects of prenatal care upon the health of the newborn. Am J Public Health 1979a;69:653–660.

Gortmacher S. Poverty and infant mortality in the United States. Am Sociol Rev 1979b;44:280–297.

Greenberg R. The impact of prenatal care in different social groups. Am J Obstet Gynecol 1983;145:797–801.

Harris J. Prenatal medical care and infant mortality. In: Fuchs V, ed. Economic aspects of health. Chicago: University of Chicago Press, 1982:15–52.

Hemminki E, Starfield B. Prevention of low birth weight and preterm birth. Milbank Mem Fund Q/Health & Society 1978;56:339–61.

Hicks L, Langham R, Takenaka J. Cognitive and health measures following early nutritional supplementation: a sibling study. Am J Public Health 1982;72:1110–18.

Kennedy E, Gershoff S, Reed R, Austin J. Evaluation of the effect of WIC supplemental feeding on birth weight. J Am Diet Assoc 1982;80:220–27.

Kessner D. Infant death: an analysis by maternal risk and health care. Washington, D.C.: Institute of Medicine, National Academy of Sciences, 1973.

Lanman J, Kohl S, Bedell J. Changes in pregnancy outcome after liberalization of the New York State abortion law. Am J Obstet Gynecol 1974;118:485–92.

Levy B, Wilkinson F, Marine W. Reducing neonatal mortality rate with nurse-midwives. Am J Obstet Gynecol 1971;109:50–58.

Lewit E. The demand for prenatal care and the production of healthy infants. In: Sirageldin I, Salkever D, Sorkin A, eds. The demand for prenatal care and the production of healthy infants, vol. 3. Greenwich, Conn.: JAI Press, 1983.

Maternal & Child Health Services. Promoting the health of mothers and children. FY 1973:30–31. (Cited in Davis & Schoen, op. cit., p. 140.)

Morris N, Udry J, Chase C. Shifting age-parity distribution of births and the decrease in infant mortality. Am J Public Health 1975;65:359–62.

NCHS (National Center for Health Statistics). Infant mortality rates: socioeconomic factors. United States. Vital Health Stat, series 22, no. 14, 1972a (DHEW publication no. (HSM)72-1045).

NCHS (National Center for Health Statistics). Trends in prematurity, United States 1950–67. Vital Health Stat, series 3, no. 15, 1972b (DHEW publication no. (HSM)72-1030).

NCHS (National Center for Health Statistics). Prenatal care: United States 1969–1975. Vital Health Stat, series 21, no. 33, 1978 (DHEW publication no. (PHS)78-1911).

NCHS (National Center for Health Statistics). Final natality statistics, 1977. Advance report. Mon Vital Stat Rep, vol. 27, no. 11, suppl., 1979 (DHEW publication no. (PHS)79-1120).

NCHS (National Center for Health Statistics). Factors associated with low birth weight, U.S., 1976. Vital Health Stat, series 21, no. 37, 1980a (DHEW publication no. (PHS)80-1915).

NCHS (National Center for Health Statistics). Final natality statistics, 1978. Advance report. Mon Vital Stat Rep, vol. 29, no. 1, suppl., 1980b (DHHS publication no. (PHS)80-1120).

NCHS (National Center for Health Statistics). Advance report of final natality statistics, 1979. Mon Vital Stat Rep, vol. 30, no. 2, suppl. (2), 1981.

NCHS (National Center for Health Statistics). Advance report of final natality statistics, 1980. Mon Vital Stat Rep, vol. 31, no. 8, suppl., 1982.

NCHS (National Center for Health Statistics). Health, United States, 1983, and prevention profile. Washington, D.C.: U.S. Govt. Printing Office, 1983 (DHHS publication no. (PHS)84-1232).

Pakter J, Nelson F. Factors in the unprecedented decline in infant mortality in New York City. Bull NY Acad Med 1974;50:839-68.

Peoples M, Siegel E. Measuring the impact of programs for mothers and infants on prenatal care and low birth weight: the value of refined analysis. Med Care 1983;21:586-605.

Placek P. Maternal and infant health factors associated with low infant birth weight: findings from the 1972 national natality survey. In: Reed D, Stanley F, eds. The epidemiology of prematurity. Baltimore: Urban & Schwarzenberg, 1977:197-212.

Prentice A, Watkinson M, Whitehead R, Lamb W, Cole T. Prenatal dietary supplementation of African women and birth weight. Lancet 1983;no. 8323:489-91.

Pritchard J, Whalley P. High-risk pregnancy and reproductive outcome. In: Gluck L, ed. Modern perinatal medicine. Chicago: Yearbook Medical Publishers, 1974:111-20.

Quick J, Greenlick M, Roghmann K. Prenatal care and pregnancy outcome in an HMO and general population: a multivariate cohort analysis. Am J Public Health 1982;71:381-90.

Rantakallio P. Social background of mothers who smoke during pregnancy and influence of these factors on the offspring. Soc Sci Med 1979;13A:423-29.

Rush D, Stein Z, Susser M. A randomized controlled trial of prenatal nutritional supplementation in New York City. Pediatrics 1980;65:683-97.

Shah F, Abbey H. Effects of some factors on neonatal and postneonatal mortality. Milbank Mem Fund Q 1971;49:33-57.

Shapiro S. New reductions in infant mortality: the challenge of low birth weight. Am J Public Health 1981;71:365-66.

Shapiro S, McCormick M, Starfield B, Krischer J, Bross D. Relevance of correlates of infant deaths for significant morbidity at one year of age. Am J Obstet Gynecol 1980;136:363-73.

Shapiro S, Schlesinger E, Nesbitt R. Infant, perinatal, maternal, and childhood mortality in the United States. Cambridge, Mass.: Harvard University Press, 1968.

Showstack J, Budetti P, Minkler D. Determiners of birthweight: the role of prenatal medical care and other factors. Am J Public Health 1984;74:1003-8.

Sokol R, Woolf R, Rosen M, Weingarden K. Risk, antepartum care, and outcomes: impact of a maternity and infant care project. Obstet Gynecol 1980;56:150-56.

Tayback M, Entwisle G, Hebel J, Hess M, McDill M, Rottman C, Young

M. Evaluation studies on maternal and infant care projects: final report. College Park, Md.: University of Maryland, 1973.

USGAO (U.S. General Accounting Office). WIC evaluations provide some favorable but no conclusive evidence on the effects expected for the special supplemental program for women, infants, and children. January 30, 1984. GAO/PEMD-84-4.

5
Teenage Childbearing

Barbara Starfield

Teenagers and their children are at increased risk of health problems both during pregnancy and afterward, so teenage childbearing is a medical as well as social concern (Chilman 1980). The proportion of infants who are of low birth weight (under 2,501 grams) is substantially higher among offspring of young mothers: 14.6 percent at under 15 years, 12.1 percent for 15 year olds, 10.7 percent for 16 year olds, 10.0 percent for 17 year olds, 9.4 percent for 18 year olds, 8.4 percent for 19 year olds, 6.9 percent for 20–24 year olds, and 5.8 percent for 25–29 year olds. Even the relatively elevated low birth weight frequency at age 45–49 (9.2 percent) is lower than that for mothers under 18 (NCHS 1982b). Infant mortality is higher in offspring of teenagers, in both the neonatal and postneonatal periods (Menken 1980; Shapiro et al. 1980), and there is greater long-term health and developmental disadvantage to children of teenagers (Furstenberg 1976; Baldwin and Cain 1980; Jekel et al. 1975; McCormick et al. 1984). Teenage mothers who become pregnant are more likely to drop out of school than other teenagers (Moore 1978; Furstenberg et al. 1981; Card and Wise 1978). Moreover, early first births are associated with increased subsequent childbearing (Trussell and Menken 1980).

Contrary to widespread belief, rates of births to teenagers have fallen markedly since 1950. Except for an upward trend from 1952 to 1957 (the "baby boom" years) and an even smaller increase in the late 1960s, the trend was continually downward until 1976, when the rate leveled (NCHS 1982a, 2). Table 3 indicates that this downward trend was limited to births in wedlock; the birth rate of unmarried teenagers has increased steadily. (This may be, in part, a reflection of greater acceptance of nonwed mothers with a larger proportion of pregnant women opting for unmarried status over time.)

Teenagers are far more likely than older women to rely upon governmental support for their deliveries. Data from Rhode Island (Dryfoos 1980) show that 69 percent of births to females under age 15, 46 percent at 15–19 years old, and 14 percent at age 20 or older are paid for from public funds,

Table 3
Selected Natality Indicators for Women under 20, United States, 1950–80

	1950	1955	1960	1965	1970	1975	1977	1979	1980
BIRTHRATES									
All women (per 1,000)									
15–19	81.6	90.3	89.1	70.4	68.3	56.3	53.7	53.4	53.0
18–19	—	—	—	—	114.7	85.7	81.9	81.3	82.1
15–17	—	—	—	—	38.8	36.6	34.5	32.3	32.5
<15	1.0	0.9	0.8	0.8	1.2	1.3	1.2	1.2	1.1
Married women (per 1,000)									
15–19	410.4	460.2	530.6	462.3	443.7	315.8	—	—	—
Unmarried women (per 1,000)									
15–19	12.6	15.1	15.3	16.7	22.4	24.2	25.5	26.9	27.6
18–19	—	—	—	—	32.9	32.8	35.0	37.2	39.0
15–17	—	—	—	—	17.1	19.5	20.7	19.9	20.6
RATIO									
Out-of-wedlock births to in-wedlock births (per 1,000 births)									
15–19	—	142	148	208	295	382	429	452	476
18–19	—	102	107	152	224	298	344	—	—
15–17	—	232	240	327	430	514	566	—	—
<15	—	663	679	785	808	870	882	—	887

Sources: NCHS 1977; NCHS 1981b; NCHS 1982b, NCHS various years.

including Medicaid and other public programs. Medicaid is the source of funding for 19 percent of deliveries to teenagers but for only 5 percent of births to women age 20 and older. However, in 1978 teenagers in this study were almost twice as likely (12.6 percent vs. 7.2 percent) as older women to have to pay the costs of delivery out of pocket. Private insurance covered the costs of delivery in only 19 percent of pregnancies of women aged under 15 and 39 percent at ages 15–19, as compared with 79 percent at ages 20 or older.

Examination of the effect of health care on teenage births is complicated because of the variety of factors that have an impact on teenage pregnancy. In contrast to the situation with many other conditions, the population at risk (sexually active females) is difficult to define, complicating the identification of suitable comparison populations for study. Examination of the impact of interventions on reducing subsequent pregnancies is fraught with methodologic problems as the risks increase both with time and with age; controlling for these effects may be difficult because of the resulting small numbers of individuals in appropriate age-risk categories. These methodologic difficulties may account at least in part for the paucity of good studies of the effectiveness of interventions. Moreover, demonstration of the impact of medical care under situations where risks are increasing because of changing social mores (as is the case for pregnancy, particularly out-of-wedlock pregnancy) is even more difficult. In these situations, constancy of the teenage birth rate may connote considerable impact of health services.

Figure 5 indicates how susceptible teenage pregnancy is to the variety of forces that impact upon it. The figure shows that the percentage of women who have borne one or more children by age 17 fluctuates, even within relatively short periods of time. Within the most recent 15 years, this percentage rose to a peak in the early 1970s and then dropped, particularly among nonwhites. Among teenagers of ages 15–19 who were interviewed in 1976, 15 percent with a prior pregnancy conceived again within a year, compared to 22 percent interviewed in 1971. (The comparable figures for repeat pregnancy within two years were 30 percent in 1976 and 50 percent in 1971 [Zelnik 1980].) Between 1972 and 1978, the total number of family planning clinic patients of ages 18 and 19 grew by about 75 percent, but the number of patients under age 17 tripled despite the decline in the total population at those ages (The Alan Guttmacher Institute 1981, 43). Of those who delayed in seeking help at a family planning clinic, approximately half appeared *after* experience with sexual intercourse; almost one-third (31 percent) indicated that the delay was due to fear that their families would find out (Zabin and Clark, unpublished data, cited in The Alan Guttmacher Institute 1981, 45).

Difficulties in determining the effectiveness of medical services are compounded by the wide variety of regulations and barriers imposed by different states and localities. National trends may mask real declines in teenage

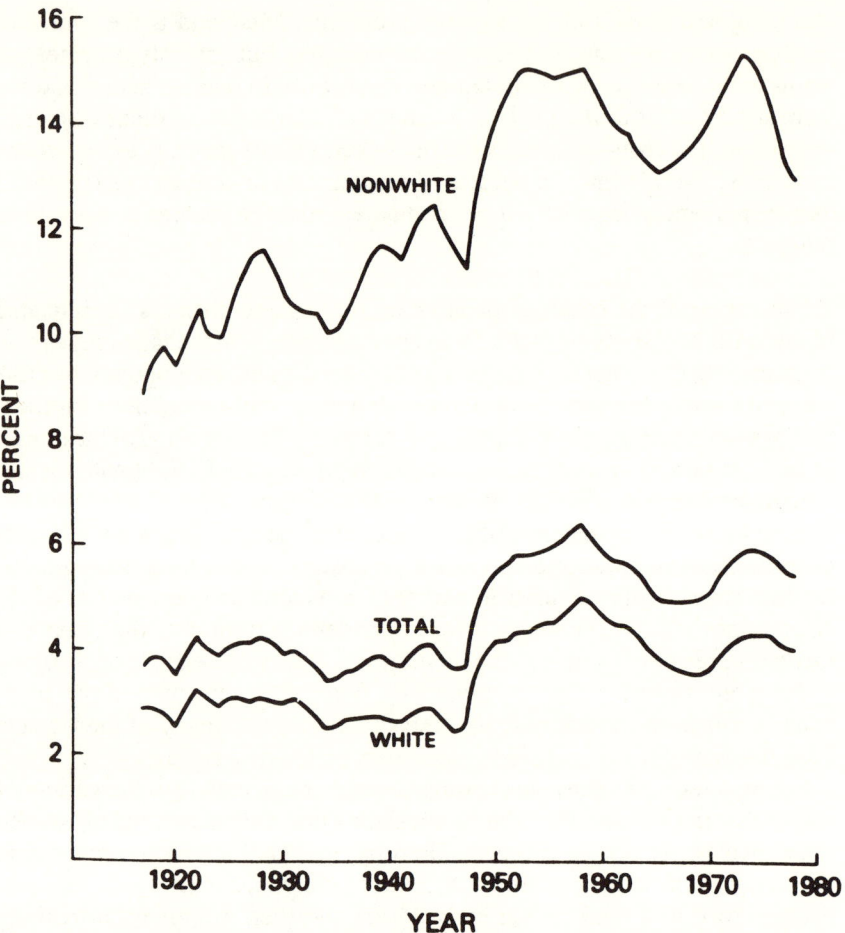

Figure 5. Percentage of Women Who Have Borne One or More Children by Age 17, by Race, United States, 1917-78
Source: Campbell 1980, 7.

pregnancies in locales where services are well developed; evaluation of the effectiveness in those locales is likely to be hampered by relatively small numbers of individuals at risk and events related to pregnancy.

As of 1981, no state had enacted a statute specifically requiring parental consent for contraception. Federal law has recognized the right to contraceptive services of minors eligible for Medicaid and AFDC federal assistance (Paul and Pilpel 1981). Despite this, about 20 percent of family planning facilities require parental consent or notification as a condition for service for patients 15 or younger; about 10 percent have such requirements for patients of ages 16-17 (Torres et al. 1980).

Despite Supreme Court rulings that women have a constitutional right (with the concurrence of their physicians) to obtain abortions (1973) and rulings that state laws which require parental consent for abortions are invalid (Paul and Pilpel 1981), some jurisdictions continue to require such consent. In 1970, 73 large cities had legal restrictions and in 28 cities length of gestation was a restriction. By 1976, only 27 cities had legal restrictions but 48 had restrictions on length of gestation (Goldstein and Wallace 1978). More than 40 percent of facilities require parental consent before providing abortion services to individuals 15 or younger; 30 percent require such consent for 16–17 year olds (Torres et al. 1980).

The impact of requirements for parental consent were demonstrated by Cartoof and Klerman (1982). In Massachusetts, requiring parental or judicial consent for minors seeking abortion was associated with a 54 percent decline in abortions among 17 year olds and a 51 percent decline among 16 year olds. The decline was greater in free-standing clinics (56 percent decline) than in hospitals (5 percent decline), and there was no decline in abortions performed by private physicians.

Prevention of pregnancy through educational programs in schools has not proved to have had much of an impact on sexual behavior (Kirby et al. 1980; Kirby 1980), with one notable exception. In that program of specialized clinics with a considerable amount of outreach and ancillary services, fertility rates dropped significantly in an uncontrolled evaluation (Edwards et al. 1980).

In contrast, the importance of family planning services, including contraception, has been demonstrated. The most effective means of contraception, "the pill" and IUDs, require medical supervision; failure rates are only 6 percent for the pill and are 12 percent for the IUD. In comparison, failure rates for the condom are 18 percent; diaphragm, 23 percent; foam, 31 percent; rhythm, 33 percent; and douche, 39 percent (Ryder 1973). The effectiveness of contraception is indicated by the fact that 62 percent of sexually active teenagers who have never used some form of birth control experienced a pregnancy as compared with 30 percent for those who have used a method inconsistently, 14 percent of those who have always used some method (including withdrawal), and 7 percent of those who have always used a medically prescribed method (pill, IUD, or diaphragm) (Zelnik and Kantner and unpublished data reported in The Alan Guttmacher Institute 1981, 15; Zelnik and Kantner 1978).

Jaffe and Dryfoos (1980) analyzed data from four sources of information: the National Reporting System for Family Planning Services (NRSFPS), which is an ongoing census of about 80 percent of the caseload of organized family planning centers; the National Ambulatory Medical Care Survey (NAMCS); the National Survey of Family Growth (NSFG), which has data on contraceptive practices and sources of care for married teenagers in 1973; and a study done at the Johns Hopkins University which provides data for all teenagers in 1971. Although it was difficult to determine the precise proportion of sexually active adolescents who received care from private physicians (because of small sample size and lack of precision in the denominator), an estimate of 15-19 percent receiving care in the private sector led the authors to estimate that 50-54 percent of the 4 million adolescents at risk in 1975 received contraceptive care from either clinics or private physicians and, of these, the number served by clinics was greater than the number served by private physicians. Thus, facilities in the public or quasi public sphere are much more involved in issues surrounding teenage pregnancy than is the case for most other conditions. About 40 percent of the 5,000 organized family planning facilities are served by health departments, 30 percent by Planned Parenthood, 19 percent by other community and neighborhood agencies, and 11 percent by hospitals (The Alan Guttmacher Institute 1981, 43).

Data from family planning clinics from 1973 to 1975 indicate that about half of the adolescent patients used no method of contraception prior to enrollment and in 1974 and 1975 an additional one-sixth used nonmedical methods. At the last clinic visit studied, approximately five-sixths reported using either the pill or an IUD. In contrast, less than one-fifth of patients aged 20-29 used no method prior to enrollment and 14 percent used the least effective methods. By 1978, 75 percent were using the pill and 4 percent an IUD according to unpublished tabulations from an NRSFPS survey in 1978 (cited in The Alan Guttmacher Institute 1981, 44). Thus, family planning clinics accomplish two functions: they serve as the only source of contraceptive care for a large proportion of teenagers at risk for pregnancy and they upgrade the practices of others from less to more effective methods (Jaffe and Dryfoos 1980).

Between 1971 and 1976, the proportion of teenagers practicing contraception increased from 18 to 30 percent; those using contraception at the last intercourse increased from 54 to 64 percent. Of those who were using contraception in 1976, 47 percent were using the pill, 21 percent the condom, 17 percent withdrawal, 3 percent an IUD, and 8 percent other methods (Zelnik and Kantner 1977).

The experiences in two adjacent counties in California, Humboldt and Del Norte, is instructive. In Humboldt County, state and federal family planning funds increased from $79,867 in 1975 to $468,188 in 1980 and $614,647 in 1981. From 1975 to 1980 the number of subsidized family planning visits increased from 2,981 to 13,921. Although the abortion rates and the teenage pregnancy rates declined only slightly in that period, they climbed in neighboring Del Norte County, which has minimal access to low-cost contraceptive services and no "family-life" or sex education program (McKeegan 1982).

Reviews of a few specific programs to prevent teenage pregnancies have concluded that teenagers feel positively about the programs. Benefits with regard to enhanced continuation of schooling have not been uniform but most of the few well-conducted evaluations have found that subsequent fertility is reduced (Klerman 1979; CDC 1980). For example one study published in 1972 found that approximately 50 percent of participants were pregnant again by 26 months as contrasted with 66 percent in the comparison group (Currie et al. 1972).

More recent evaluations suggest somewhat greater benefit than earlier studies (CDC 1980). In a very comprehensive program that is school-oriented but located outside the school in St. Paul, Minnesota, there were no repeat pregnancies through 1978 (the program was initiated in 1973) and the fertility rate fell significantly: from 79 births per 1,000 female students in 1972-73 to 35 per 1,000 in 1975-76 (Edwards et al. 1977). In western Massachusetts, there was a decline in the pregnancy rate of more than 50 percent attributable to a sexuality/contraceptive awareness program; after the program was discontinued in 1976 the pregnancy rate rose. The Centers for Disease Control 1980 concluded that the benefits of these programs were a result of their effectiveness in preventing pregnancy by encouraging contraception, because the programs also reduced the abortion rate.

In the country as a whole, however, there is little doubt that the availability of abortions has been associated with declines in birth rates among teenagers. Although slightly under 20 percent of the childbearing population is under age 20, teenagers accounted for one-third of all abortions in 1979 (calculations from data in NCHS 1982a). This overrepresentation of teenagers has been present at least since abortion was legalized; in 1973, 30 percent of legal abortions were performed on the 17 percent of females under age 20 and the trend persisted throughout the 1970s. (NCHS 1981b; NCHS 1981a, table 12). The data would be even more striking if rates of abortion were calculated only for teenagers who are sexually active and therefore at risk of pregnancy. Between 1968 and 1973 the number and rate of abortions in teenagers increased (CDC Abortion Surveillance Annual Summaries, 1973-79). By 1975, 36 percent of all pregnancies among teenagers were terminated by abortion compared with 22 percent among women aged 20-24 (Jaffe and Dryfoos 1980).

Abortion services are provided disproportionately to the nonpoor, even though poor teenagers have higher pregnancy rates. In a study in Rhode Island, 56 percent of pregnancies occurring in teenagers living in high socioeconomic (SES) areas and 42 percent of pregnancies in teenagers in middle SES areas ended in abortion, as compared with 28 percent in low SES areas and 22 percent in poverty areas (Dryfoos cited in The Alan Guttmacher Institute 1981, 52). About 90 percent of teenagers who obtain abortions get them in free-standing clinics rather than hospitals (Lindheim 1979).

In Atlanta, Georgia, an array of free-standing first-trimester abortion clinics were established and two hospitals accelerated their provision of abortion services in 1973. This was followed, in 1974, by a decline in the fertility of young adolescents (ages 10-14), a group that had experienced a markedly disproportionate increase in fertility in the decade before that with especially rapidly increasing rates from 1970 to 1973. The decline in rate was much greater for white teenagers than for nonwhites, and was much greater in central Atlanta than in suburban Atlanta, other urban areas, or the remainder of the state. Evidence suggesting that these differences were due to differences in access to care derive from data on the timing of abortions; for black teenagers under age 15 the proportion of abortions done in the second or third trimester was 19 percent (compared with 7.3 percent for all abortions in Georgia); among black teenagers outside of central Atlanta 24.7 percent of abortions were after the first trimester (Shelton 1977).

Only 23 percent of U.S. counties have any facility providing abortions; services are particularly sparse in nonmetropolitan areas (The Alan Guttmacher Institute 1981, 54). Fifty-five percent of teenagers who obtain abortions travel to other counties to get them, partly because of lack of availability of resources nearby and partly because of state counterparts of Hyde amendment restrictions on public-funding of abortions in some states (Torres et al. 1980). Teenagers are more likely to have delayed abortions than older women. Only one third of abortions in teenagers under age 15 are performed at less than nine weeks' gestation compared with 41 percent among 15-19 year olds and 51 percent at ages 10-24 (The Alan Guttmacher Institute 1981, 55).

Despite the unevenness in availability of abortion facilities and the barriers imposed by requirements for parental consent, abortions have reduced the frequency of births to teenagers. Moreover, since its legalization, abortion has been associated with decreased subsequent pregnancy rates: teenagers whose first pregnancy ended in abortion were only half as likely (9.9 percent) to become pregnant a second time within the following year than those whose pregnancy resulted in a live birth (17.5 percent) (Zelnik 1980). Rates of pregnancy per 1,000 sexually active females have declined since the early 1970s, particularly among 15-17 year olds (The Alan Guttmacher Institute 1981, Figure 12, p. 19). Overall, birth rates fell abruptly in all age groups in the early 1970s and have continued to fall in all age groups (NCHS 1982a). The decline for teenagers is all the more noteworthy because of increasing sexual activity among that group (Furstenberg et al, 1981, 1-17).

Thus, despite the difficulties in conducting studies to assess the impact of health services in reducing births to teenagers, there is substantial evidence of the effectiveness of both family planning services and the availability of abortions.

References

The Alan Guttmacher Institute. Teenage pregnancy: the problem that hasn't gone away. New York, 1981.

Baldwin W, Cain V. The children of teenage parents. Fam Plann Perspect 1980;12:34–43.

Campbell A. Trends in teenage childbearing in the United States. In: Chilman, op. cit., 1980:3–13.

Card J, Wise L. Teenage mothers and teenage fathers: the impact of early

childbearing on the parents' personal and professional lives. Fam Plann Perspect 1978;10:199-205.
Cartoof V, Klerman L. Massachusetts' parental consent law: a preliminary study of the law's effects. Mass J Community Health 1982;14-19.
CDC (Centers for Disease Control). Successful programs to prevent pregnancy in adolescents. MMWR Jan. 18, 1980; 29(2):15-21.
Chilman C. Adolescent pregnancy and childbearing: findings from research. Washington, D.C., December 1980 (USDHHS (PHS) NIH publication no. 81-2077).
Currie J, Jekel J, Klerman L. Subsequent pregnancies among teenage mothers enrolled in a special program. Am J Public Health 1972;62:1606-11.
Dryfoos J. Adolescent pregnancy in Rhode Island: report to the Rhode Island Health Services Research, Inc., 1980 (contract no. HRA 232-78-0089 no. VRP 10).
Edwards L, Steinman M, Arnold K, Hakanson E. Adolescent pregnancy prevention services in high school clinics. Fam Plann Perspect 1980;12:6-14.
Edwards L, Steinman M, Hakanson E. An experimental comprehensive high school clinic. Am J Public Health 1977;67:765-66.
Furstenberg F. Unplanned parenthood: the social consequences of teenage childbearing. New York: Free Press, 1976.
Furstenberg F, Lincoln R, Menken J. Teenage sexuality, pregnancy, and childbearing. Philadelphia: University of Pennsylvania Press, 1981:7-8.
Goldstein H, Wallace H. Services for and needs of pregnant teenagers in large cities of the United States, 1976. Public Health Rep 1978;93:46-54.
Holtzman N. The goal of preventing early death. In: Blendon R, Duval M, Hiscock W, eds. Conditions for change in the health system. USDHEW Public Health Service, Washington, D.C.: U.S. Government Printing Office, 1977:107-32. (DHEW publication no.(HRA)78-642).
Jaffe F, Dryfoos J. Fertility control services for adolescents: access and utilization. In: Chilman, op. cit., 1980:129-56.
Jekel J, Harrison J, Bancroft D, Tyler N, Klerman L. A comparison of the health of index and subsequent babies born to school age mothers. Am J Public Health 1975;65:370-74.
Kirby D. The effects of school sex education programs: a review of the literature. J Sch Health 1980;50:559-63.
Kirby D, Alter J, Scales P. An analysis of U.S. sex education programs and evaluation methods. Springfield, Va.: National Technical Information Service, vols. I-V, 1980, (DHEW report no. CDC-2021-79-DK-FR-1).
Klerman L. Evaluating service programs for school-age parents: design problems. In R. Barker Bausell (ed) Evaluation and the health professions, vol. 2. Beverly Hills, Ca.: Sage Publications, 1979:55-70.
Lindheim B. Services, policies, and costs in U.S. abortion facilities. Fam Plann Perspect 1979;11:283.

McCormick M, Shapiro S, Starfield B. High-risk young mothers: infant mortality and morbidity in four areas in the United States 1973-1978. Am J Public Health 1984;74:18-23.

McKeegan M. Teenage pregnancy in Humboldt County: critiquing a critic. Fam Plann Perspect 1982;14:339-40.

Menken J. The health and demographic consequences of adolescent pregnancy and childbearing. In: Chilman, op. cit., 1980:177-205.

Moore, K. The consequences of age at first childbirth: educational attainment. Washington, D.C.: Urban Institute Press, 1978. U.S. Dept. of Commerce PB 289051 (NTIS).

NCHS (National Center for Health Statistics). Natality Statistics. Teenage childbearing: United States, 1966-75. Mon Vital Stat Rep, vol. 26, no. 5 (suppl.), 1977.

NCHS (National Center for Health Statistics). Induced terminations of pregnancy: reporting states 1977 and 1978. Mon Vital Stat Rep, vol. 30, no. 6 (suppl.), Sept. 28, 1981a.

NCHS (National Center for Health Statistics). Advance report of final natality statistics 1979. Mon Vital Stat Rep, vol. 30, no. 6 (suppl.), Sept. 29, 1981b, table 12.

NCHS (National Center for Health Statistics). Induced terminations of pregnancy: reporting states 1979. Mon Vital Stat Rep, vol. 31, no. 7 (suppl.), Oct. 25, 1982a.

NCHS (National Center for Health Statistics). Advance report of final natality statistics 1980. Mon Vital Stat Rep, vol. 31, no. 8 (suppl.), Nov. 30, 1982b.

NCHS (National Center for Health Statistics). Vital Statistics, Vol. 1 for various years.

Paul E, Pilpel H. Teenagers and pregnancy: the law in 1979. In: Furstenberg, Lincoln, Menken, op. cit., 1981:409-19.

Ryder N. Contraceptive failure in the U.S. Fam Plann Perspect 1973; 5:133-42.

Shapiro S, McCormick M, Starfield B, Krischer J, Bross D. Relevance of correlates of infant deaths for significant morbidity at one year of age. Am J Obstet Gynecol 1980;136:363-73.

Shelton J. Very young adolescent women in Georgia: has abortion or contraception lowered their fertility? Am J Public Health 1977;67:616-20.

Torres A, Forrest J, Eisman S. Telling parents: clinic policies and adolescents' use of family planning and abortion services. Fam Plann Perspect 1980;12:284.

Trussell J, Menken J. Early childbearing and subsequent fertility. In: Furstenberg, Lincoln, Menken, op. cit., 1981:234-50.

Zelnik M. Second pregnancies to premaritally pregnant teenagers 1976 and 1971. Fam Plann Perspect 1980;12:69.

Zelnik M, Kantner J. Sexual and contraceptive experience of young unmarried women in the United States 1976 and 1971. Fam Plann Perspect 1977;9:55-56, 58-63, 67-71.

Zelnik M, Kantner J. Contraceptive patterns and premarital pregnancy among women aged 15-19 in 1976. Fam Plann Perspect 1978;10:135.

Zelnik M, Kantner J. Sexual activity, contraceptive use, and pregnancy among metropolitan-area teenagers 1971-1979. Fam Plann Perspect 1980;12:230.

6
Inadequate Immunization and the Prevention of Communicable Diseases

Lisa Egbuonu and Barbara Starfield

Immunization has markedly decreased morbidity and mortality from vaccine-preventable communicable disease. Poliomyelitis has been almost completely eliminated: paralytic cases declined from 18,308 in 1954 to 6 in 1981 (CDC 1982a, 12, 15) (Figure 6). Measles cases declined from 385,158 cases/year in 1963 (when measles vaccine was licensed) to 3,124 in 1981 (CDC 1982b, 12, 14) (Figure 7). This has resulted in a decline in measles encephalitis and measles-related deaths (CDC 1977, 7-13). Pertussis declined from more than 60,000 cases/year in the mid 1950s, when pertussis immunization (vaccine) became standardized, to 1,248 cases in 1981 (CDC 1982a, 12, 15). Declines in pertussis-related deaths paralleled the decrease in reported cases (CDC 1982a) (Figure 8). Reported cases of rubella and congenital rubella also declined after rubella vaccine was licensed in 1969 (CDC 1982a, 12-14) (Figure 9). Similarly, there has been a decrease in mumps, tetanus (and tetanus-related deaths), and diphtheria (and diphtheria-related deaths) (CDC 1982a, 32, 62, 87).

Despite the obvious benefits of immunization in decreasing morbidity and mortality from common childhood infectious diseases, large gaps in immunization coverage remain. Surveys in 1977 indicated that 20 percent of children aged 0-13 years were inadequately immunized against diphtheria, pertussis, and tetanus (Krugman and Katz 1977); among children aged 1-4, 40 percent were not fully immunized against polio, 30 percent were inadequately immunized against diphtheria, pertussis, and tetanus, 37 percent were not immunized against measles, and 41 percent were not immunized against rubella (Marks et al. 1979). As a result, an Immunization Initiative was begun in 1977 by the federal government with the aim of raising the level of immunization to greater than 90 percent among school children. By

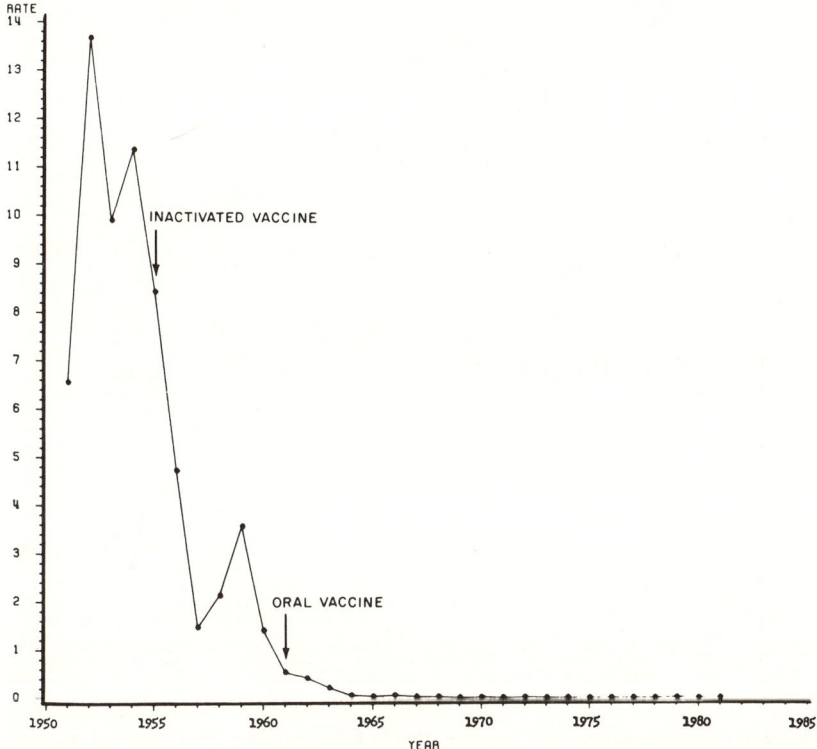

Figure 6. Reported Cases of Poliomyelitis (Paralytic) per 100,000 Population, by Year, United States, 1951–81
Source: CDC 1982a, 69.

1979 immunization levels of students in kindergarten through twelfth grade for diphtheria, pertussis, tetanus, polio, and measles were reported as at or above 90 percent, rubella levels were at 83 percent, and mumps immunization levels were 58 percent. Levels were even higher for children entering school in the fall of 1978: over 90 percent for DPT, polio, measles, and rubella and 83 percent for mumps (Hinman and Preblud 1980). For the school year 1980/81 the proportion of children immunized upon entry to kindergarten or first grade was reported to be more than 95 percent for measles, rubella, polio, and DPT and 91 percent for mumps (CDC 1980).

There is evidence that the immunization rates as reported by the Centers for Disease Control overestimate the immunization status of children. Immunization surveys conducted among school-age children (1980–82) in rural North Dakota, small-town Colorado, and urban New York indicated that at every site the immunization levels reported by state officials to CDC exceeded the levels found in the school survey (usually by 7–10 percent). This survey (DeAngelis et al. 1983) involved extensive follow-up of records and avoided procedures that in some studies led to overreporting of incom-

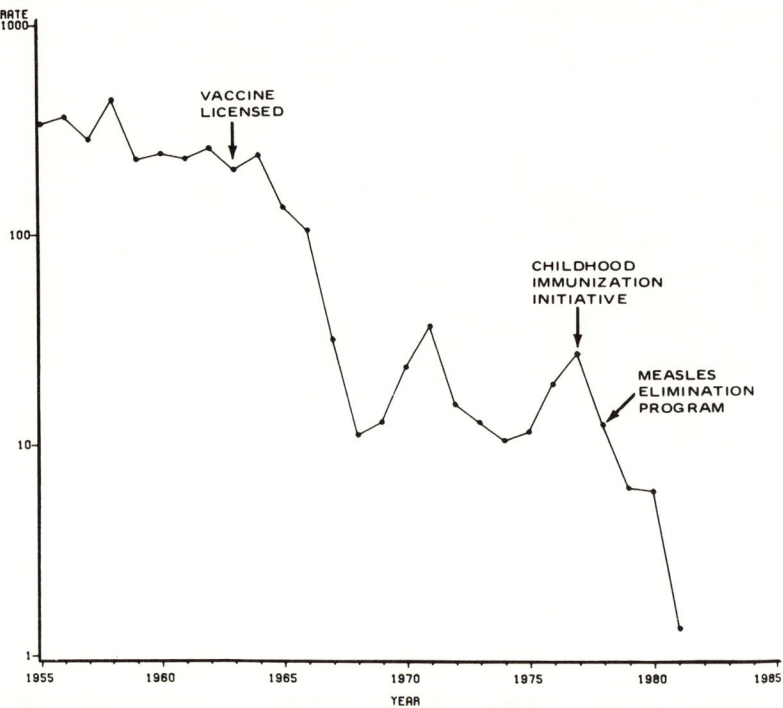

Figure 7. Reported Cases of Measles (Rubeola) per 100,000 Population, by Year, United States, 1955–81
Source: CDC 1982a, 54.

plete vaccinations due to difficulties in obtaining accurate information (Gottlieb 1976).

Second, the estimate that more than 90 percent of school-age children are immunized for each specific disease does not adequately reflect the percentage of children who are not fully immunized against all seven. For example, in 1980/81 in California more than 90 percent of children entering kindergarten or first grade were immunized against each of the seven diseases but the percentage immunized against all seven was only 77 percent. In some states, the percentage was considerably lower. For example, only 54 percent of children entering kindergarten or first grade in Arizona were immunized against all seven diseases (CDC 1980). Unfortunately not all states report the percent immunized against all seven diseases and therefore a true national weighted average cannot be computed.

Third, the data concern only school-age children. Immunization is required for school entry in all states and there is no requirement for immunizations in the preschool age period except for children enrolled in facilities such as day care. Data from the Maryland Health Department Immunization Survey indicate that, in 1980, 45 percent of two-year old children were inadequately immunized (three DPTs); 56 percent did not have the four DPT

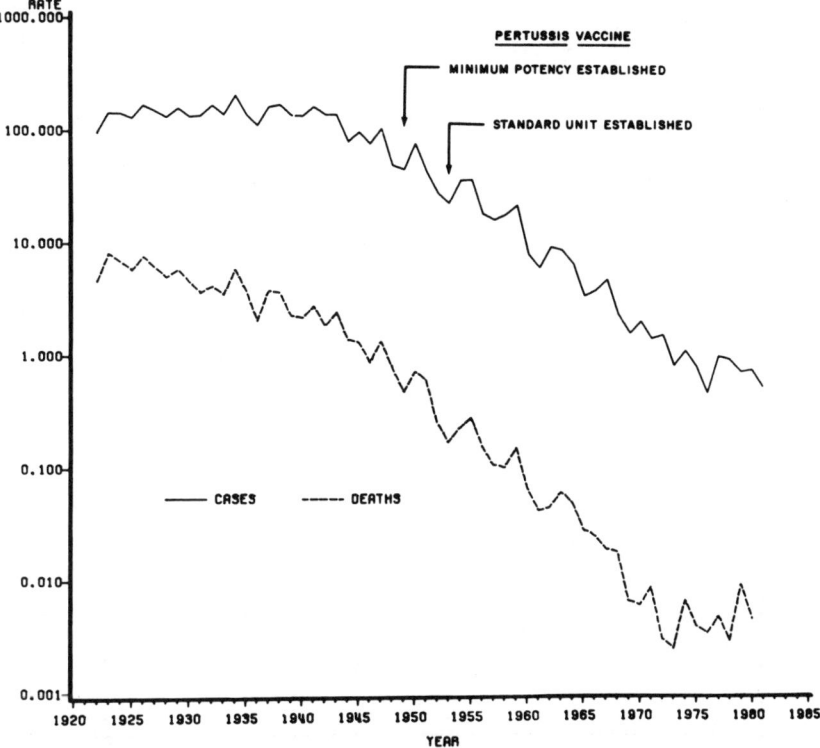

Figure 8. Reported Cases of Pertussis (Whooping Cough) and Deaths per 100,000 Population, by Year, United States, 1922-81
Source: CDC 1982a, 65.

immunizations required for optimal immunity (C Jones, personal communication). Data from Ohio indicate that, in 1977, 28 percent were inadequately immunized even when mumps immunization was excluded from the definition of complete immunization (Ohio Dept. of Health 1978); 60 percent were inadequately immunized if mumps and a fourth DPT were included in the criterion (Marks et al. 1979).

Moreover, immunization coverage is particularly low in certain segments of the population, i.e., in poverty areas and among nonwhite children. A study conducted in 1977 among children attending a neighborhood health center from Roxbury and Dorchester (predominantly minority and poor) showed that only 22 percent of children aged 19-23 months were fully immunized (Minear and Guyer 1979). A study of two year olds in Ohio in 1977 showed that low paternal and maternal education, low socioeconomic status, and large family size were associated with increased risk of incomplete immunizations (Marks et al. 1979).

Adolescents and young adults are also at high risk of disease because of inadequate immunization. Many individuals in these age groups were not

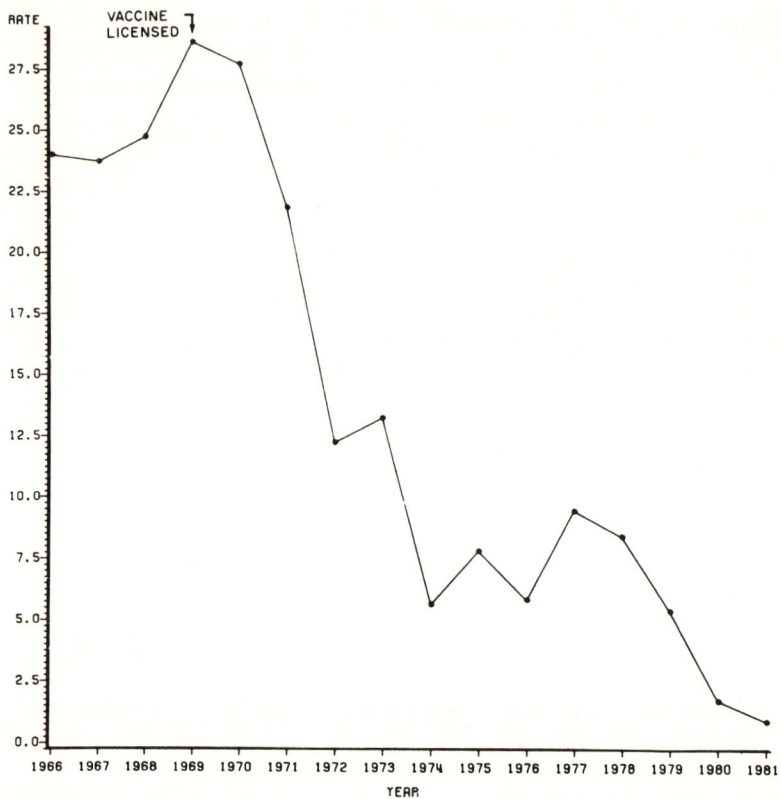

Figure 9. Reported Cases of Rubella (German Measles) per 100,000 Population, by Year, United States, 1966-81
Source: CDC 1982a, 74.

adequately immunized as children yet were not exposed to disease and resulting "natural immunity" because of relatively high overall levels of immunization among their peers. This group has periodic outbreaks of measles and rubella (vide infra).

In summary, large numbers of children continue to be inadequately immunized—including school-age children, preschoolers, poor and minority children, and adolescents.

Inadequate immunization produces an ever-present threat of recurrence of epidemics. The pertussis experience in England and Wales demonstrates that a drop in immunization coverage can lead to the reappearance of epidemics. Pertussis vaccine began to be widely used in 1958. From 1958–74, 75 percent of children were immunized against pertussis by two years of age. The number of reported cases dropped by 66 percent from 1957 to 1961. Following controversy concerning the adverse reactions to pertussis vaccine, immunization levels dropped from 77 percent in 1974 to 30 percent in 1978. A large outbreak of pertussis occurred in 1978–79 (CDC 1982c, 629–

32). Rates of reported cases were highest in districts with the lowest immunization coverage (Pollard 1980). Age-specific incidence rates rose most sharply among children under four years of age (who had very low immunization coverage) and least sharply among children 5–9 years of age (who had been vaccinated prior to the vaccine controversy). Vaccine efficacy was 93 percent. The 1977–79 epidemic is estimated to have caused the hospital admission of 5,000 children (2,000 of these less than six months old); approximately 50 children required intensive care, 200 had pneumonia, and 83 had convulsions. Children under one year of age had a case fatality rate of 0.19 per 100 reported cases and accounted for 71 percent of the pertussis-related deaths. After the 1977–79 outbreak, vaccine coverage increased to 45 percent in 1981 but another even larger epidemic, the largest since 1957, occurred in 1981–82 (CDC 1982c). The importance of maintaining high levels of immunization against pertussis is clear.

In the United States pertussis outbreaks continue to occur. Atlanta experienced one in 1977 and Maryland had one in 1982. Of 41 cases reported in Maryland in August 1977, 36 (88 percent) had received fewer than three doses of DPT. Seventeen were not properly immunized; of these only two were the result of parental refusal of vaccine because of fear of side effects. The majority of the remainder were due to illness at the time vaccine was to be given with no subsequent follow-up; other reasons were frequent moving, prematurity, or lack of knowledge of the importance of immunization (Buck et al. 1982a). By the end of November, 61 cases had been reported in Maryland for 1982 (Buck et al. 1982b).

Another continuing problem is posed by the persistence of congenital rubella. Rubella is usually a mild illness. The principal reason for vaccination is to prevent the development of spontaneous abortions and congenital rubella syndrome, which occur when the fetus is exposed to maternal rubella in the first trimester of pregnancy. Common sequelae of intrauterine infection are cardiac lesions, eye defects (especially cataracts), deafness, growth retardation, and central nervous system defects. The last nationwide epidemic of rubella occurred in 1964 and resulted in 20,000 cases of congenital rubella syndrome. Following the licensing of vaccine in 1969, federal programs and funds were directed toward disseminating the vaccine to children. The rationale was that immunizing children would interrupt the transmission of the disease in the community and thus decrease the likelihood of exposure and infection of pregnant women. As a result of the emphasis on immunization coverage for children, disease incidence decreased mainly among those under 15 years of age (Hinman and Preblud 1980; Hinman 1982). Studies in California showed that, relative to the antibody levels in the population attained by natural infection (1968–69), rubella immunization markedly increased antibody levels in children but had much less effect on antibody levels in teenagers and adults (Dales and Chin 1982). Outbreaks continued to occur in junior and senior high schools and colleges. Rubella epidemics occurring in Chicago in 1978 caused 31 cases of congenital rubella syndrome (Lamprecht et al. 1982). Epidemics also occurred in Seattle in 1981, at the University of Southern California in 1981, and at the University of California at Berkeley in 1981 (Hinman 1982). The incidence of rubella among women of childbearing age remained high and congenital rubella syndrome declined at a much slower rate than did rubella (Hinman 1982). The frequency of reported rubella began to drop sharply among 15-19 year olds in 1980, probably due to better enforcement of school immunization laws and as a result of immunization of these adolescents when they were toddlers (Hinman 1982). However, continued efforts are needed to increase immunization levels for women of childbearing age and to maintain high levels of immunity among children in order to further decrease congenital rubella syndrome.

McDaniel and colleagues (1975) found that children receiving care exclusively from health departments had higher immunization levels than those who received care exclusively from private practitioners, but the poorest coverage was found in children who received care from both health department and private practitioners, suggesting that continuity of care is an important determinant of immunization completeness. A study by the Ohio Department of Health (1978), however, indicated that patients of private practitioners had better immunization levels than those receiving care from public clinics even after socioeconomic status was controlled. Gordis and Markowitz (1971) found that patients receiving comprehensive care and traditional care did not differ in the completeness of their immunizations, although the patients studied were all high risk and may have received more follow-up than the general population. Immunization levels have been shown to be higher when patients keep their own immunization records (McCormick et al. 1981). These studies indicate that there is no clear evidence that the site of care, per se, has a determining influence on immunization levels.

In contrast, the relationship between the availability of public funds for immunization and disease incidence is very clear. Mumps immunization, which has often not been included among publicly funded programs, has never reached levels near those of the other six diseases (Hinman and Preblud 1980; CDC 1980). The Immunization Initiative of 1977 (which consisted of increased federal support for immunization) increased public education, increased cooperation between government agencies, and facilitated enactment and enforcement of school immunization laws. This resulted in a major increase in vaccine administration in the public sector, a significant increase in immunization coverage, and decrease in morbidity due to vaccine-preventable diseases (Hinman and Preblud 1980). The clearest example of the direct relationship between federal funds, immunization programs, and increased immunization levels and decreased disease incidence was seen in the case of measles.

Measles vaccine was licensed in 1963. At the annual meeting of the

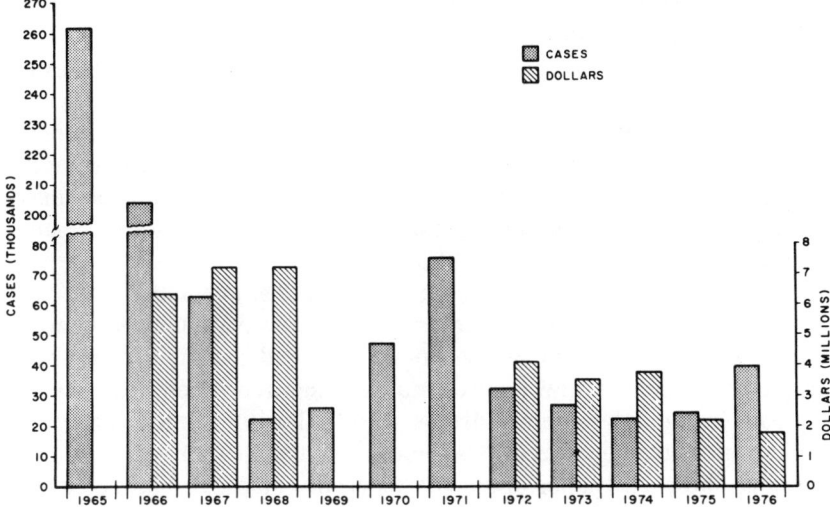

Figure 10. Measles Cases* and Federal Grant Funds** Obligated for Measles Control Programs, by Year, United States, 1965–76
Source: CDC 1977, 2.
* Per calendar year
**Per fiscal year

American Public Health Association in 1966, it was announced that the epidemiologic basis for eradication of measles existed in the United States. During the next three years large amounts of federal funds were spent on measles immunization. The number of reported cases dropped to 22,231 in 1968 (Hinman 1982). However, from 1969 to 1971 the licensing of rubella vaccine led to a shift in federal funds away from measles immunization (Hinman 1982). Many states lacked funds to purchase measles vaccine and many health departments stopped vaccination efforts (Witte and Axnick 1975). This resulted in a decrease in the number of doses of vaccines distributed and an increase in the number of measles cases and deaths (CDC 1977, 1–15). Federal funds for measles immunization were reinstated in 1971 and the number of cases declined in 1972. The importance of federal support is shown in Figure 10.

In 1976 and 1977 an upsurge in the number of measles cases occurred as a result of vaccine failures among those immunized under 12 months of age and among those immunized with killed measles vaccine, and as a result of the low level of immunization coverage in the 10–13 year age group (only 67 percent vaccinated against measles). As a result of the Immunization Initiative and the Centers for Disease Control campaign to eradicate measles (initiated in 1978), both of which involved federal funds, immunization levels increased to 90 percent for school children in 1978. The overall incidence of measles decreased, particularly in the 10-14 year age group; in 1981 the highest age-specific incidence was in children under five.

Children under five accounted for 31 percent of the reported cases of measles in 1981. The majority (52 percent) of these cases under age five were in children over 15 months of age who were not attending nursery school or day care centers (which have mandatory immunization coverage). Children under 15 months of age (too young for immunization) accounted for 40 percent of the cases and those attending nursery or day care centers accounted for 8 percent (Hinman 1982).

In addition, measles epidemics continue to occur among individuals over 15 years of age. Many in this age group were never immunized or were unsuccessfully immunized but had never acquired the disease naturally since most of their cohort was successfully immunized. There were several outbreaks in high schools and colleges in 1981 and 1982 although reported immunization coverage was over 90 percent (Hinman 1982).

Despite these continuing problems especially among preschoolers not attending a day care center or nursery school and adolescents and young adults, in 1982 the centralized federally funded measles eradication campaign attained the lowest rate of measles cases in recorded history (CDC 1982b).

Disease morbidity and mortality has been dramatically decreased by immunization. When immunization coverage decreased, disease incidence increased. The availability and amount of federal funds for immunization are inversely related to inadequate immunization and disease incidence. Continuing public support of surveillance and targeting of immunizations to high-risk groups is essential to prevent a resurgence of vaccine-preventable diseases.

References

Buck C, Pitts J, Israel E. Pertussis outbreak in Maryland 1982. State of Maryland Division of Communicable Diseases and Epidemiology Newsletter, September, 1982a.

Buck C, Pitts J, Israel E. Pertussis outbreak update. State of Maryland Division of Communicable Diseases and Epidemiology Newsletter, November, 1982b.

CDC (Centers for Disease Control). Measles surveillance report no. 10, 1973-76. Centers for Disease Control, July, 1977.

CDC (Centers for Disease Control). School year immunization data 1980-81, special tabulation, 1980.

CDC (Centers for Disease Control). Annual summary 1981: reported morbidity and mortality in the United States. MMWR 1982a;30(54).

CDC (Centers for Disease Control). Elimination of indigenous measles—United States. MMWR Oct. 1, 1982b;31(38):517-19.

CDC (Centers for Disease Control). Pertussis—England and Wales. MMWR Dec. 3, 1982c;31(47):629-32.
Dales L, Chin J. Public health implications of rubella antibody levels in California. Am J Public Health 1982;72(2):167-72.
DeAngelis C, Berman B, Oda D, Meeker R. Achieving optimal immunization levels in school-age children: what are the necessary ingredients? J Pediatr 1983;103:811-14.
Fulginiti VA, ed. Immunization in clinical practice. Philadelphia: JB Lippincott, 1982.
Gottlieb N, Wechsler H. Immunization levels in Boston schools: a second look. N Engl J Med 1976;294:1459-61.
Gordis L, Markowitz M. Evaluation of the effectiveness of comprehensive and continuous pediatric care. Pediatrics 1971;48:766-76.
Hinman AR. Measles and rubella in adolescents and young adults. Hosp Pract 1982;17:137-49.
Hinman AR, Preblud SR. Epidemic potential of measles and rubella. J Am Coll Health Assoc 1980;29:105-9.
Krugman S, Katz S. Childhood immunization procedures. JAMA 1977;237:2228-30.
Lamprecht C, Schauf V, Warren D, Nelson K, Northrop R, Christiansen M. An outbreak of congenital rubella in Chicago. JAMA 1982;247:1129-33.
McCormick M, Shapiro S, Starfield B. The association of patient-held records and completion of immunizations. Clin Pediatr 1981;20:270-74.
McDaniel D, Patton E, Mather J. Immunization activities of private-practice physicians: a record audit. Pediatrics 1975;56:504-7.
Marks J, Alpin T, Irvin J, Johnson D, Keller J. Risk factors associated with failure to receive vaccinations. Pediatrics 1979;64:304-9.
Minear R, Guyer B. Assessing immunization services at a neighborhood health center. Pediatrics 1979;63:416-19.
Ohio Department of Health. Ohio immunization level survey of two-year-old children April-July 1977. Columbus: Ohio Department of Health, 1978.
Pollard R. Relation between vaccination and notification rates for whooping cough in England and Wales. Lancet 1980;1:1180-82.
Witte J, Axnick M. The benefits from 10 years of measles immunization in the United States. Public Health Rep 1975;90:205-7.

7
Acute Rheumatic Fever

Barbara Starfield

Acute rheumatic fever (ARF) is thought to be a disease in the process of disappearing. By the late 1970s, the incidence of ARF was about 1.8 episodes per 100,000 persons per year. Although there are wide geographic variations in incidence (Pantell 1981), the decline has been under way for decades, even preceding the use of antibiotics (Pantell 1981).

A variety of studies document the decline in occurrence of rheumatic fever over the past five decades, although none compile the data in a way that permits the association of changes in medical care delivery with changes in the rate of decline. Quinn and colleagues (Quinn et al. 1970; Quinn and Federspiel 1974) showed the importance of verifying the diagnosis of rheumatic fever, both for attribution of deaths and for reported cases. Their studies in Nashville showed a generally declining yearly incidence rate (per 100,000 population) of rheumatic fever from 1964 through 1969 as follows: 12.8 in 1963, 14.9 in 1964, 10.0 in 1965, 10.2 in 1966, 11.3 in 1967, 6.4 in 1968, and 8.2 in 1969.

A comparison of data from the National Health Survey from 1935–36 and data from Baltimore in 1960–64 and 1968–70 indicates a decline in incidence of both initial and recurrent attacks of rheumatic fever, with a greater drop in recurrent attacks. In Baltimore, incidence rates per 100,000 children ages 5–14 were 20.9 in 1960–64 and 13.5 in 1968–70 (Gordis 1980).

Annegers et al. (1982) demonstrated declining incidence rates in four separate areas: Malmö, Sweden; Connecticut; Nashville, Tennessee, and Rochester, Minnesota (Figure 11). Quinn et al. (1970) demonstrated a decline in verified death rates from 1940 to 1965. Death rates were persistently higher among individuals in the lower social classes than in the higher social classes, and the disparity in death rates between the lower and upper social classes was greater in 1956–65 than in 1940–45 (before effective therapy) (Quinn et al. 1970). The rate of decline in death rates from 1940 to 1964 in the United States was greater for deaths from acute rheumatic fever than for deaths from chronic rheumatic heart disease (Acheson 1965).

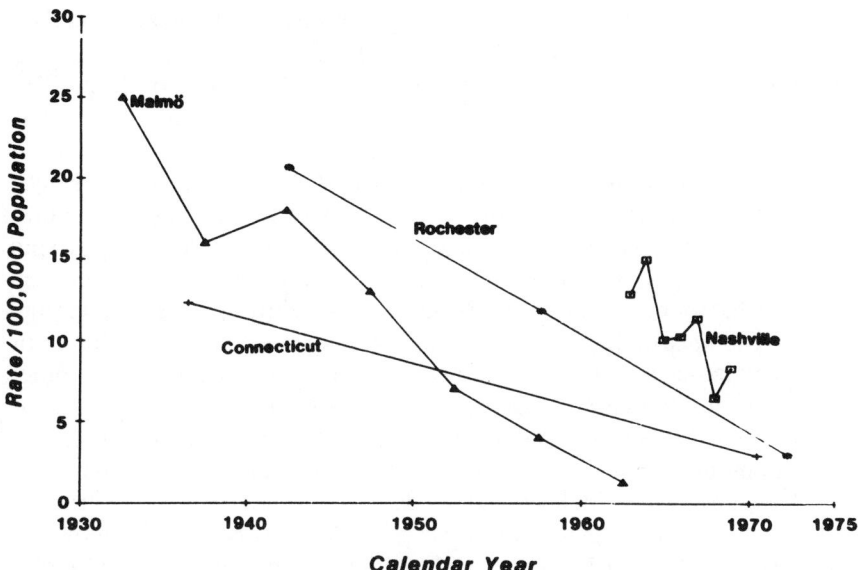

Figure 11. Incidence of Rheumatic Fever in Four Studies: Malmö, Sweden; Connecticut; Rochester, Minnesota; and Nashville, Tennessee
Source: Annegers et al. 1982, 756.

The theoretical basis for a beneficial effect of medical care derives from the fact that ARF is associated with infection (usually symptomatic pharyngitis) by the beta-hemolytic streptococcus, an organism sensitive to antibiotics. Moreover, detection of the organism in individuals with pharyngitis is possible using a throat culture.

Treatment of infection with group A beta-hemolytic streptococcus reduces the likelihood of occurrence of a new case of ARF, i.e., primary ARF (Denny et al. 1950); prophylactic antibiotics reduce the likelihood of recurrences of ARF in individuals previously diagnosed as having ARF (Spagnuolo et al. 1971). The magnitude of the reduction in occurrence of primary ARF by treatment with parenteral penicillin is eightfold to tenfold (Denny et al. 1950). In a study of the efficacy of various types of antibiotics in preventing recurrences of ARF, Spagnuolo et al. (1971) found that the relative risk of recurrence was greater for individuals receiving oral penicillin or sulfadizine than for those receiving parenteral (intramuscular) penicillin.

Rapid therapy of individuals with streptococcal illness is associated with lower secondary attack rates. Among 464 children treated with antibiotics within 48 hours of onset the secondary attack rate among siblings was 16.1 percent, whereas in 156 patients treated after 48 hours the attack rate was 34.6 percent (Breese and Disney 1956). Thus, rapid treatment reduces the pool of individuals potentially susceptible to ARF.

The risk of ARF in individuals who have had a prior attack is much greater than in individuals never before having ARF (Tompkins et al. 1977), and the attack rate in patients with two or more prior attacks is higher than in those with only one prior attack (Spagnuolo et al. 1971). Therefore, at least theoretically, receipt of care from providers who are aware of the patient's history should facilitate more appropriate management of individuals with pharyngitis among the susceptible population.

Although individuals with prior attacks of ARF are clearly a vulnerable population because they are at increased risk of recurrences, identification of those susceptible to first attacks is difficult. Pharyngitis, and even streptococcal pharyngitis, is extremely common in childhood. Pantell (1981) calculated that for every 100,000 persons, 30,000 yearly episodes of pharyngitis and 5,000 episodes of streptococcal pharyngitis occur. Moreover, of the 5,000 streptococcal infections, only 2,500 are truly infectious; the others reflect carrier states that do not predispose to ARF. The maximum attack rate of ARF is 1.5 episodes of rheumatic fever per 1,000 untreated streptococcal infections under nonepidemic conditions (Pantell 1981). At least two analyses have provided guidelines on the cost-effectiveness of various strategies to detect individuals potentially susceptible to primary ARF (Tompkins et al. 1977; Pantell 1981). Both conclude that it is cost-effective to obtain a throat culture for individuals with symptomatic pharyngitis (except in epidemic situations where treatment without culture is warranted). In one of the analyses (not limited to pediatric patients), the disadvantages of diagnostic workup and therapy were calculated to outweigh the potential benefits when the community prevalence of infection is less than 5 percent. It should be noted that in most geographic areas, the community prevalence of the organism is between the lower figure of 5 percent and the epidemic rate (30 percent).

Effectiveness of medical care in preventing ARF can therefore derive from three types of interventions: the availability of efficacious preventive therapies, the facilitation of access to medical care for earlier diagnosis and treatment of streptococcal pharyngitis, and better ongoing care for the prophylaxis of recurrent streptococcal illness.

Evidence suggesting an impact of medical care of all three types is provided by declines of both primary and recurrent ARF coincident with the widespread availability of antibiotics and certain important changes in the health care system. Before antibiotics were available, 60 to 70 percent of rheumatic subjects had one or more recurrences (Roth et al. 1937). Markowitz and Gordis (1972) reported that with preventive measures approximately 5 percent of patients on oral prophylaxis (and less than 1 percent on parenteral penicillin) have recurrences. In Rochester, Minnesota, the Epidemiology Program Project provided community prevalence rates that included both nonhospitalized as well as hospitalized individuals. Cases not hospitalized accounted for 30 percent in the 1935-49 period, 15 percent during 1950-64, and 19 percent in 1965-78. The age-adjusted incidence rate per 100,000 population for initial attacks fell from 13.6 in 1935-49 to 8.2 in 1950-64 (a decline of 41 percent) to 2.7 in 1965–78 (a decline of 67 percent). Rates for recurrent attacks declined even more, from 7.0 to 3.2 (a 54 percent decline) to 0.3 (a 91 percent decline) over the same three time periods. (Well over half of the cases in all periods were children or teenagers and the decline was seen at all ages. For children of ages 5–14 [the peak ages of occurrence] the incidence rates were 65, 41, and 9, respectively.) The first time period roughly corresponded to the preantibiotic era (except for 1945–49) and the last time period to the era after access to medical care was greatly improved (1965).

A demonstration of the actual effectiveness of medical care was provided by a study of Gordis (1973). In this study, the incidence of hospitalized first attacks of rheumatic fever in children ages 5–14 was determined for the periods 1960–64 and 1968–70 in groups of census tracts ("eligible tracts") served by comprehensive child health care programs that were initiated in the mid-1960s, and comparison groups of census tracts without such programs ("not eligible tracts"). In 1960–64 the incidence rates were greater in the eligible tracts (26.8 per 100,000) than in the comparison tracts (18.1 in tracts adjacent to the eligible tracts, 8.1 in nonadjacent tracts, and 14.6 in nonadjacent tracts similar in racial characteristics to the eligible tracts). In 1968–70, subsequent to the development of the health care programs, the rates were lower (10.6) in the eligible tracts—a 60 percent decline—than in the other tracts (15.3, 14.6, and 14.9, respectively). Moreover, in 1960–64, 30 percent of the children had no prior history of respiratory infection whereas the comparable figure for 1968–70 was 48 percent; the decline in incidence in the city (accounted for entirely by the decline in the eligible tracts) was limited to individuals with a prior respiratory infection. That is, children for whom medical care would not have been sought because they had no symptoms preceding ARF had no decline in incidence of ARF, whereas the incidence in children whose symptoms would likely have prompted medical care halved. Further (although indirect) evidence that the effect was due to medical care was provided by the observation that 80 percent of all throat cultures processed by the state laboratory were from patients residing in eligible tracts. Also, surveys in the community showed that over 95 percent of eligible children were, in fact, registered in the comprehensive care programs. These results provide firm evidence that the theoretical benefit of medical care in preventing ARF are, in fact, realized in areas that provide care which is organized to adequately recognize, diagnose, and manage situations that are a threat to health.

Despite the remarkable decline in frequency of occurrence, the persistence of acute rheumatic fever in particular subgroups of the population suggests that medical care still has an important role in control of ARF. Land and Bisno (1983) reported that the overall incidence of acute rheumatic fever in Memphis-Shelby County (Tennessee) was 0.64 cases per 100,000 population per year during 1977–81. In this community-based study that included both hospitalized (as determined by review of hospital records) and nonhospitalized cases (as reported in a mail survey of family physicians, internists, pediatricians, and neurologists), the incidence rates were much greater for blacks than for whites. Moreover, the incidence rates were much greater in families living in inner city (poorer) areas than in suburban and rural areas, both among whites and blacks.

References

Acheson R. The epidemiology of acute rheumatic fever 1950-64. J Chronic Dis 1965;18:723-24.

Annegers J, Pillman N, Weidman W, Kurland L. Rheumatic fever in Rochester, Minnesota, 1935-1978. Mayo Clin Proc 1982;57:753-57.

Breese B, Disney F. Factors influencing the spread of beta hemolytic streptococcal infections within the family group. Pediatrics 1956;17:834-41.

Denny FW, Wannamaker LW, Brink WR, Rammelkamp CH, Custer EA. Prevention of rheumatic fever. JAMA 1950;143:151-53.

Gordis L. Effectiveness of comprehensive-care programs in preventing rheumatic fever. N Engl J Med 1973;289:331-35.

Gordis L. Streptococcal disease. In: Last J, ed. Public health and preventive medicine. 11th ed. New York: Appleton-Century-Crofts, 1980:173-85.

Land M, Bisno A. Acute rheumatic fever: a vanishing disease in suburbia. JAMA 1983;249:895-98.

Markowitz M, Gordis L. Rheumatic fever. Philadelphia: W.B. Saunders, 1972.

Pantell R. Pharyngitis: diagnosis and management. Pediatrics in Review 1981;3:35-39.

Quinn R, Federspiel C. The incidence of rheumatic fever in metropolitan Nashville, 1963-1969. Am J Epidemiol 1974;99:273-80.

Quinn R, Sprague H, Quinn J. Mortality rates for rheumatic fever and rheumatic heart disease, 1940-65. Public Health Rep 1970;85:1091-1101.

Roth IR, Ling C, Whittemore A. Heart disease in children: a rheumatic group. I. Certain aspects of the age of onset and of recurrences in 488 cases of juvenile rheumatism ushered in by major clinical manifestations. Amer Heart J 1937;13:36-60.

Siegel AC, Johnson EE, Stollerman GH. Controlled studies of streptococcal pharyngitis in a pediatric population. 1. Factors related to attack rate of rheumatic fever. N Engl J Med 1961;265:559-66.

Spagnuolo M, Pasternack B, Tranta A. Risk of rheumatic fever recurrences after streptococcal infection. N Engl J Med 1971;285:641-47.

Tompkins R, Burnes D, Cable W. An analysis of the cost effectiveness of pharyngitis management and acute rheumatic fever prevention. Ann Intern Med 1977;86:481-92.

8
Child Battering (Abuse)

Lawrence S. Wissow and Barbara Starfield

Abuse is an important cause of injury and death among children. In 1976, 60,000 children per year were estimated to suffer significant physical injury, including 2,000 with fatal injuries and 6,000 with permanent central nervous system injury (Kempe 1976). Between 1 and 7 percent of children brought to medical care may have experienced abuse or neglect (Altemeir et al. 1982; Helfer 1982), although they all are not diagnosed as such. Abuse reports and the number of deaths attributed to abuse are increasing (Jason et al. 1982, Maryland, State of, 1982), and there is historic as well as epidemiologic evidence that worsening economic conditions and unemployment are related to increases in child deprivation and abuse. On the basis of survey data, Margolis and Farran (1984) estimated that children in a family where the father is unemployed incur a threefold increase in risk of being abused compared with other children.

The mandate for medical involvement in issues related to child abuse is inescapable. Laws requiring reports of suspected abuse are nearly universal in the United States, and the courts have found health care workers to be responsible for taking measures to protect potential victims of abuse (Curran 1977; Newberger and Hyde 1975). A moral imperative for medical care involvement exists; prospective studies of "untreated" abuse find that more than half of abused children will be victims again or will suffer permanent residua and that the severity of abuse increases with time from the initial incident (Hamory and Jeffreys 1977; Friedman 1972).

Attempts to prevent child abuse may be of the primary or secondary type. Primary action is aimed at preventing abuse before it occurs; secondary intervention prevents further, more serious, abuse once an episode has come to medical attention. Prevention is based on the premise that mistreatment is caused by maladaptive responses to the stresses of parenthood, rather than by true malicious feeling for the child. The sources of poor adaptation may be many; some parents may have social, emotional, and intellectual handicaps that antedate the birth of their children. Parents who themselves were abused, for example, appear to be at a higher risk of becoming abusers. For others, childbirth brings with it changes in family and financial status that may cause stress. The child's temperament may also play a role, testing the patience and coping skills of even the most devoted parents (Newberger and Hyde 1975). Many workers believe that programs can be created to help parents improve their child care and coping skills.

Another presumption about cause is based upon research on nonhuman primates, which has found a critical postpartum period during which maternal-child bonding takes place. While such a critical period has not yet been demonstrated in humans, it is thought that this is the time at which mothers may be particularly in need of psychologic support to help them in the reciprocal adjustment of mother and child to each other's needs and rhythms (O'Connor et al. 1980; Hunter et al. 1978). Lack of bonding and support may reduce a mother's future ability to adjust to the emotional demands of parenthood. It should be noted that these theories and the studies that derive from them address primarily the problem of abuse in early childhood. Sexual abuse of older children is far less studied and may be much more difficult to prevent (Brassard et al. 1983; Tilelli et al. 1980).

Some clinical trials of interventions in the prenatal period or in the immediate postnatal period were well designed and yielded encouraging results (Ainsfeld et al. 1983).

Gray and coworkers (1977) used interviews, questionnaires, and observation to classify women receiving prenatal care as being at high or low risk for developing abnormal parenting practices that might lead to abuse. High- and low-risk mothers were selected for study, with the high-risk group divided into treatment and nontreatment groups of 50 each. Treatment included regular pediatric care from a single provider and weekly public health nurse home visits. The nontreatment and low-risk mothers were referred to their preferred source of care in the community. Twenty percent (5 of 25 examined in follow-up at two years) of children born to the high-risk untreated group required hospitalization for serious trauma (fractures, subdural hematoma, severe burns, ingestions), whereas there were no similar injuries in either the low-risk or treated high-risk groups.

O'Connor and coworkers (1980) conducted a trial of infant rooming-in during the postpartum hospital stay. Consecutive primagravida mothers were assigned by bed availability to rooming-in or traditional postnatal care. The rooming-in group also had a more liberal visiting policy for outside visitors (other family members). Subsequent analysis demonstrated that the groups were similar in terms of demographic characteristics and attitudes toward postnatal care. Medical records and abuse registers were searched when the children were 17 months old. Five percent (8 of 156) of the traditional care children had been hospitalized for conditions relating to parenting problems. There was only one such hospitalization among the 143 children who had roomed in. There were no differences in general measures of health status, such as immunizations, or the number of clinic visits reported for routine or acute care.

Siegel and coworkers (1980) found no statistically significant differences in hospitalization rates of children of mothers randomly assigned to traditional postpartum care as compared with those provided postpartum visiting in combination with a home health visitor, although children with traditional care were somewhat more likely to be hospitalized. Small but significant improvements in parent-child attachment were reported for those mothers who had been allowed more time with their children in the postpartum period. The amount of visiting appears to have been less than in the O'Connor study, and exclusions from the initial study population may have tended to remove those children who would have been at highest risk for abuse.

Lealman et al. (1983) also reported that the provision of more intensive posthospital care for newborns and their mothers failed to reduce the incidence of abuse and neglect. Mothers were classified into high and low risk of abuse based on medical care patterns and demographic characteristics obtained from hospital charts. Children in the intervention group were less likely to be hospitalized but were three times as likely to have failed to thrive than high-risk control group children. The study report gives only sketchy details of the intervention and the population studied. It also may be that the designation of risk by factors recorded on a hospital chart is less useful than determinations made by observation of actual parent attitudes and behavior.

Attempts at primary prevention of abuse later in childhood, and at prevention of repeated abuse (secondary prevention) have not met with notable success, although there have been no studies using a clinical trial design.

A number of demographic and psychologic factors have been associated with the occurrence of child abuse, as have a number of physical stigmata that could be noted at the time at which medical care is given. As with other conditions with fairly low prevalence, risk factors that have strong associations in retrospective studies may have very low predictive value when applied in a prospective manner (Daniel et al. 1978). These difficulties are well illustrated in the work of Rosenberg et al. (1982). The authors attempted to use risk factors (such as unkempt appearance and poor parent-child interaction) observed at the time of emergency room visits to develop a screening test for risk of abuse. Relative risks associated with the factors under study were very high, but the best predictive value that could be obtained was 42 percent, and this was achieved at a sensitivity of 15 percent. Over five times as many abuse cases were missed as were correctly identified by the screen. Poor predictive values for screening tests may be permissible where the consequences of missing a case are grave, and where the follow-up required is not costly or injurious to those falsely identified as being at risk. In the case of potential child abuse, the social risks of false labeling and the labor-intensive nature of case-finding and therapy make this sort of screening impractical (Schoeman and Reamer 1983).

Cohn (1980) evaluated 11 federally sponsored abuse intervention demonstration projects and found that 30 percent of enrolled parents committed severe, repeated abuse while under treatment; health care workers judged only 42 percent to be less likely to abuse at the end of the treatment. The 11 centers used different treatment modalities, and there were no control groups or attempts to judge comparability of patients treated at the various centers. Gabinet (1983) described a similar experience with a treatment program in Cleveland. Over half of the high-risk families contacted about treatment refused to participate, including 10 of 19 known to have previously abused their children. Of those that entered the program, more than one quarter did not give up potentially harmful behaviors. Those parents who at the onset seemed to be depressed were most helped by the program.

More drastic means of secondary prevention, i.e., those involving the separation of parents and children, show no great promise. A mainstay of secondary intervention is the use of foster care. In one state, about 15 percent of children were placed in foster care after one episode of abuse (Runyan et al. 1981). Both the way in which children are assigned to foster care and the usefulness of the practice have been questioned. Runyan and colleagues found no consistent standards that explained which children were assigned to foster families. Foster care often extends for long periods of time (sometimes measured in years) and may place children at even greater emotional and physical risk (Fanshel 1981; Markham 1980). Existing legal precedent also makes the severing of parent-child ties extremely difficult, even in the face of proven physical abuse (Santosky v. Kramer 1982). Other types of intervention, as risky as they may be for further abuse, may lead to better psychological adjustment for the child if they are successful. A longitudinal study of children, comparing those who were simply sent home with those placed in foster care or receiving intensive agency home visits suggested that intervention in the home can help family functioning and lessen further abuse (DeCastro et al. 1978). Seventeen of 21 children placed in foster care were judged to be functioning better at the end of one year although three required permanent placement. Forty-three of 69 who received agency contact in their homes improved even though most received few visits from social service personnel. Two of three children treated at home, with an intensity considered by the study authors to be adequate (20 or more visits a year), were improved. In this evaluation, however, there was no attempt to control for selection factors that determined assignment to the study groups; as these factors may also influence future behavior, the findings should be interpreted with caution.

In summary, there is evidence that serious trauma and abuse are prevented by measures begun in the prenatal or early postnatal period and aimed at promoting better parent-child relationships early in life. Although this evidence is limited by the small size of the groups of parents observed, the restriction of the studies to particular institutions or programs, and the relatively short periods of follow-up, the findings of the several studies are consistent, in contrast to the findings of studies involving later primary prevention or prevention of recurrence. As abuse is an uncommon (although important) condition, efforts to identify individuals at risk will result in a large number of individuals falsely identified, even with a method that has a relatively high sensitivity and high specificity. Therefore, ethical considerations alone suggest that preventive measures should be applied to all parents rather than just those thought to be at risk. Interventions in the context of medical care provided before or soon after birth are more consistently fruitful than the social services and family therapy that have been employed in risk reduction programs for families of older infants and children and those who are already victims of abuse.

References

Ainsfeld E, Curry MA, Hales DJ, et al. Maternal-infant bonding: a joint rebuttal. Pediatrics 1983;72:569-71.

Altemeir WA, O'Connor S, Vietze PM, Sandler HM, Sherrod KB. Antecedents of child abuse. J Pediatr 1982;100:823-29.

Brassard MR, Tyler AH, Kehle TJ. School programs to prevent intrafamilial child sexual abuse. Child Abuse Negl 1983;7:241-45.

Cohn AH. The pediatrician's role in the treatment of child abuse: implications from a national evaluation study. Pediatrics 1980;65:358-60.

Curran WJ. Failure to diagnose battered child syndrome. N Engl J Med 1977;296:795-96.

Daniel JH, Newberger EH, Reed RB, Kotelchuck M. Child abuse screening—implications of the limited predictive power of abuse discriminants from a controlled family study of pediatric social illness. Child Abuse Negl 1978;2:247-59.

DeCastro FJ, Rolfe UT, Heppe M. Child abuse, an operational longitudinal study. Child Abuse Negl 1978;2:51-55.

Fanshel D. Decision making under uncertainty: foster care for abused children. Am J Public Health 1981;71:685-86.

Friedman SB. The need for intensive follow-up of abused children. In: Kempe CH, Helfer RE, eds. Helping the battered child and his family. Philadelphia: J.B. Lippincott, 1972.

Gabinet L. Child abuse treatment failures reveal need for redefinition of the problem. Child Abuse Negl 1983;7:395-402.

Gray JD, Cutler CA, Dean JG, Kempe CH. Prediction and prevention of child abuse and neglect. Child Abuse Negl 1977;1:45-58.

Hamory J, Jeffreys M. Flexibility and innovation in multidisciplinary management of child abuse in western Australia. Child Abuse Negl 1977;1:217-39.

Helfer RE. A review of the literature on the prevention of child abuse and neglect. Child Abuse Negl 1982;6:251-61.

Hunter RS, Kilstrom N, Kraybill EN, Loda F. Antecedents of child abuse and neglect in premature infants: a prospective study in a newborn intensive care unit. Pediatrics 1978;61:629–35.

Jason J, Andereck ND, Marks J, Tyler CW. Child abuse in Georgia: a method to evaluate risk factors and reporting bias. Am J Public Health 1982;72:1353–58.

Kempe CH. Approaches to preventing child abuse. Am J Dis Child 1976;130:941–47.

Lealman GT, Phillips JM, Haigh D, Stone J, Ord-Smith C. Prediction and prevention of child abuse—an empty hope? Lancet 1983;1:1423–24.

Margolis LH, Farran DC. Unemployment and children. Int J Mental Health 1984;13:107–24.

Markham B. Child abuse intervention: conflicts in current practice and legal theory. Pediatrics 1980;65:180–85.

Maryland, State of, Social Services Administration. Annual summary of suspected child abuse reports received (manuscript 1982).

Newberger EH, Hyde JN. Child abuse: principles and implications of current pediatric practice. Pediatr Clin North Am 1975;22:695–715.

O'Connor S, Vietze PM, Sherrod KB, Sandler HM, Altemeir WA. Reduced incidence of parenting inadequacy following rooming in. Pediatrics 1980;66:176–82.

Rosenberg NM, Meyers S, Shackleton N. Prediction of child abuse in an ambulatory setting. Pediatrics 1982;70:879–82.

Runyan DK, Gould CL, Trost DC, Lado FA. Determinants of foster care placements for the maltreated child. Am J Public Health 1981;71:706–11.

Santosky v. Kramer, no. 80-5889. Fam Law Reporter 1982;8:3023–25.

Schoeman F, Reamer FG. Should child abuse always be reported? Hastings Cent Rep 1983;13(4):19–20.

Siegel E, Bauman KE, Schaefer ES, Saunders MN, Ingram DD. Hospital and home support during infancy: impact on maternal attachment, child abuse and neglect, and health care utilization. Pediatrics 1980;66:183–90.

Tilelli JA, Turek D, Jaffe AC. Sexual abuse of children. N Engl J Med 1980;302:319–23.

Part II

Child Health Problems Amenable to Prevention by Medical Care through Detection and Management in the Premorbid Stage

9
Congenital Hypothyroidism and Phenylketonuria

Lisa Egbuonu and Barbara Starfield

Screening of newborns for congenital hypothyroidism and phenylketonuria with subsequent diagnosis and management of affected infants is important in the prevention of mental retardation. The incidence of congenital hypothyroidism is approximately 1 per 4,000 live births (LaFranchi et al. 1979; Fisher et al. 1979). The incidence of phenylketonuria is 1 in 15,000 live births (Holtzman et al. 1974).

Each of these conditions results in severe morbidity if untreated. Congenital hypothyroidism results in mental and growth retardation if left untreated (Frost et al. 1979; Raiti and Newns 1971). Without treatment one third require special schools and one fourth have an IQ under 70 (Hulse et al. 1980). Infants treated before the age of three months have a good prognosis; most have IQs above 90 (Frost et al. 1979, Raiti and Newns 1971, Klein et al. 1972). Unfortunately, diagnosis based on clinical signs and symptoms is difficult and often is delayed past the time that treatment is most effective (Klein et al. 1972; Frost et al. 1979). In one large screening program carried out at 4–8 weeks of age only 2.9 percent of infants diagnosed as congenitally hypothyroid by screening were suspected of having hypothyroidism on clinical grounds. Evidence indicates that infants treated in the program, all of whom received therapy by eight weeks of age, had normal development (Fisher et al. 1979). Thus congenital hypothyroidism is a fairly common disease in which early diagnosis and treatment is essential for good prognosis; early diagnosis requires screening of the newborn infant.

Newborn screening is of equal importance in the prevention of phenylketonuria. Without screening, phenylketonuria is usually not detected until irreversible mental retardation has occurred. Early diagnosis and treatment with a phenylalanine-restricted diet results in normal IQ scores for almost all children with phenylketonuria (Williamson et al. 1981; Dobson et al. 1977;

Wrona 1979). Neonatal screening, diagnosis, and treatment are essential in preventing mental retardation from this disease.

Procedures to confirm diagnoses for infants with a positive screening test are accurate and relatively simple. A wide network of well-known facilities, all of them based in tertiary medical institutions, perform these tests and serve as referral centers for the prescription and supervision of a very efficacious intervention. This intervention consists of a diet low in phenylalanine, which must be maintained by the affected individual at least through the first few years of life. Both diagnosis and treatment strategies are of well-documented efficacy; the general excellence of follow-up and supervision and financial support for families that cannot afford the special foods is responsible for good compliance with the regimen (Williamson et al. 1981). Therefore, the main concern is the adequacy of the screening process that detects infants at risk.

The importance of organizational factors in achieving effectiveness of screening was indicated by an international comparative study in the United States, United Kingdom, and Ireland in 1973 (Starfield and Holtzman 1975).

In the United Kingdom, infants are tested at an optimal time (between 6 and 14 days of age). If infants have left the hospital before this time, screening becomes the responsibility of the local health authority. Blood specimens are obtained by personnel who must visit all infants in their homes by two weeks of age. Delay in follow-up testing is minimal because channels of communication between the procurer of the specimen, the laboratory, local public health personnel, consultants, and practitioners are clearly defined. The specimen is sent to a designated laboratory; abnormal test results are reported immediately to the local authority (which arranges for either hospitalization or a repeat test depending on the results of the initial test). The general practitioner has responsibility for the primary care of the children, with consultation from a tertiary care center in the region. The mean duration of time between screening and follow-up is seven days (with a standard deviation of seven days).

In Ireland, screening is done earlier than the optimum age, which results in a failure to recognize some affected infants. However, there is very rapid institution of follow-up and treatment (mean number of days between screening and follow-up is five, with a standard deviation of five days). There is only one screening laboratory and lines of communication between the laboratory, local public health personnel, and consultative personnel are well established.

In the United States, in contrast, in many states several laboratories may perform the tests, and there is evidence of marked variation in quality (Holtzman et al. 1974). Due to poor lines of communication in many areas, the mean number of days between screening and follow-up is 12 (with a large standard deviation of 19 days, undoubtedly reflecting great variability in effectiveness of the screening process) (Starfield and Holtzman 1975).

Although the adequacy of screening for hypothyroidism has not been as extensively studied as that for phenylketonuria, studies in at least one area suggest the importance of organizational features of the program. In a five-year period (1976-80), inadequacies in the screening program resulted in missed diagnoses in 19 of 159 affected infants (12 percent) in New England. Three infants were not screened, six infants had their diagnoses missed because of errors in the processing of the specimens, five infants were tested before elevations in thyroid stimulating hormone occurred, and in five infants diagnosis and/or treatment was delayed. Descriptions of the reasons for at least some of these failures indicate the importance of a centralized responsibility for monitoring the entire process from taking the initial specimen to institution of therapy. Procedures that were instituted after the study resulted in marked improvement in effectiveness of screening. These procedures included written instructions regarding responsibility for obtaining the initial specimen, monitoring of procedures in laboratories, and apprising parents in writing of the need to repeat screening tests (Report of the New England Regional Screening Program and the New England Congenital Hypothyroidism Collaborative 1982).

As of October 1980, all 50 states and Washington, D.C., had newborn screening programs; 48 had legislative statutes for the program (the remaining 3 had regulations promulgated by the respective departments of health). Conditions amenable to screening, and covered by many of these states' laws, include homocystinuria, galactosemia, maple syrup urine disease, tyrosinemia, and sickle cell anemia. But by far the most common conditions for which newborn screening is mandated by law are phenylketonuria and hypothyroidism. In 1980, 48 states required screening for phenylketonuria and 41 required screening for hypothyroidism (National Clearinghouse for Human Genetic Disease 1981).

Data from 49 states and the District of Columbia in 1974 indicated that 16 states (32 percent) were providing free tests. States that provided free tests were more likely to have centralized testing. The state lab was the only lab conducting the tests in 5 of the 16 states providing free tests (31 percent); in contrast the state lab was the only facility providing the tests in 4 of the 36 states not providing free tests (11 percent) (Committee for the Study of Inborn Errors of Metabolism 1975). Thus, states that provide the test without charge were more likely to have centralized services. Although more recent data on the relationship between the method of paying for the lab tests and centralization of laboratories is not available, it is known that more states were providing free tests in 1982 than in 1974. A survey sent to officials in all states in 1982 resulted in 38 responses. Of these, 15 states charged for the screening test; of the 23 states that did not, 8 were contemplating doing so (Holtzman 1983). It is possible that the institution of a charge by public laboratories will result in more tests being done in private commercial and hospital labs. This raises several concerns about the effectiveness of screening programs in the future.

There is a general consensus that centralized laboratories are more accurate and efficient for neonatal screening (Brandon 1980; Committee on Genetics 1982). The American Academy of Pediatrics recommends that analysis of samples be centralized in order to enhance evaluation of efficiency, accuracy, participation, and adequacy of samples; accuracy is improved with high volumes of samples per unit of time (Committee on Genetics 1982). Commercial and hospital laboratories miss detecting phenylketonuric infants more than would be expected by the chance occurrence of false negatives (Holtzman et al. 1981; Holtzman et al. 1974). Assuring full coverage and minimizing false negatives is of vital importance in newborn screening and centralized labs do this best. In addition, decentralized small-volume operations may delay analyses until large batches can be run simultaneously. This could delay diagnosis for a variety of congenital diseases—such a delay could be fatal for infants with galactosemia and maple syrup urine disease (which occur in 1 in 50,000 to 1 in 150,000 live births) (Holtzman et al. 1981) and serious for infants with conditions such as hypothyroidism and phenylketonuria. Finally, follow-up of positive screening tests requires confirmation of diagnosis and treatment; this is best done with a centralized screening facility and the resources to coordinate follow-up (Brandon 1980; Holtzman 1981; Fisher et al. 1979).

In summary, congenital hypothyroidism and phenylketonuria are not uncommon conditions that are amenable to treatment. Early diagnosis via neonatal screening is essential and neonatal screening is best done in centralized laboratories with clear channels of communication and assumption of responsibility for follow-up. Decentralization of services, with or without withdrawal of public funding, can be expected to result in an increased number of children who are needlessly handicapped by these conditions.

References

Brandon G. Regionalization of metabolic screening laboratories. In: Bickel H, Guthrie R, Hammersen G. Neonatal screening for inborn errors of metabolism. Berlin: Springer-Verlag, 1980:275–79.

Committee for the Study of Inborn Errors of Metabolism. The development of legislation and regulation for PKU screening. In: Genetic screening: programs, principles, and research. Washington, D.C.: National Academy of Sciences, 1975:44–87.

Committee on Genetics. New issues in newborn screening for phenylketonuria and congenital hypothyroidism. Pediatrics 1982;69:104–6.

Dobson J, Williamson M, Azen C, Koch R. Intellectual assessment of 111 four-year-old children with phenylalaninemia. Pediatrics 1977;60:822–27.

Fisher D, Dussault J, Foley T, et al. Screening for congenital hypothyroidism: results of screening one million North American infants. J Pediatr 1979;94(5):700–705.

Frost G, Parkin J, Rowley D. Congenital hypothyroidism. Lancet 1979;2:1026.

Holtzman N. Newborn screening for hereditary metabolic disorders: desirable characteristics, experience, and issues. In: Kaback M ed. Genetic issues in pediatric and obstetric practice. Chicago: Year Book Medical Publishers, 1981:455–70.

Holtzman N. The impact of the federal cutback on genetic services. Am J Med Genet 1983;15:353–65.

Holtzman N, Leonard C, Farfel M. Issues in antenatal and neonatal screening and surveillance for hereditary and congenital disorders. Ann Rev Public Health 1981;2:219–51.

Holtzman N, Meek A, Mellits D. Neonatal screening for phenylketonuria. JAMA 1974;229(6):667–70.

Hulse J, Grant D, Clayton B, et al. Population screening for congenital hypothyroidism. Br Med J 1980;280:675–78.

Klein A, Meltzer S, Kenny F. Improved prognosis in congenital hypothyroidism treated before age 3 months. J Pediatr 1972;81(5):912–15.

LaFranchi S, Murphey W, Foley T, Larsen P, Buist N. Neonatal hypothyroidism detected by the northwest regional screening program. Pediatrics 1979;63(2):180–91.

National Clearinghouse for Human Genetic Disease. State laws and regulations on genetic disorders. Rockville, Maryland: Department of Health and Human Services, 1981. (publication no. (HSA)81-5243).

Raiti S, Newns G. Cretinism: early diagnosis and its relation to mental prognosis. Arch Dis Child 1971;46:692–94.

Report of the New England Regional Screening Program and the New England Congenital Hypothyroidism Collaborative. Pitfalls in screening for neonatal hypothyroidism. Pediatrics 1982;70:16–20.

Starfield B, Holtzman N. A comparison of the effectiveness of screening for phenylketonuria in the United States, United Kingdom, and Ireland. N Engl J Med 1975;293:118–21.

Williamson M, Koch R, Azen C, Chang C. Correlates of intelligence test results in treated phenylketonuric children. Pediatrics 1981;68(2):161–66.

Wrona R. A clinical epidemiologic study of hyperphenylalaninemia. Am J Public Health 1979;69(7):673–78.

10
Lead Poisoning

Mark Farfel, Nancy Hutton, and Barbara Starfield

Lead poisoning is a pervasive and persistent childhood problem in the United States. After the first U.S. case report in 1914 (Thomas and Blackfan), the number of children poisoned from lead ingestion gradually increased to the point where, in the 1930s, acute toxicity in children began to be recognized as a public health problem (Levinson and Harris 1936). The "classical" case of the 1930s, 1940s, and 1950s had acute symptoms ranging from irritability and constipation to encephalopathy and was clearly related to dilapidated slum housing with deteriorating lead-based paint and the eating of lead-containing paint chips by children (Lin-Fu 1982). Recurrence of acute toxicity after medical therapy was the rule unless the lead paint hazard was corrected and, with each recurrence, the prognosis for recovery became worse (Lin-Fu 1982).

Lead poisoning continues to be a problem in the 1980s although severe acute toxicity is now seen much less often. Poor children, particularly those who live in urban areas with old housing and heavy traffic patterns, are at highest risk. The Second National Health and Nutrition Examination Survey (1976–80) provided the first population estimates of the distribution of blood lead (PbB) levels in the general U.S. population (Mahaffey et al. 1982). The prevalence of elevated lead levels among all children 6 months to 5 years of age was 4 percent or a total of about 780,000 affected children. In that age group, 2 percent of whites, 12 percent of blacks, 2 percent of rural, 12 percent of urban, 1 percent of middle and upper class, 11 percent of poor, and 19 percent of poor, black, urban children had elevated blood lead levels as defined by the Centers for Disease Control (CDC).

All of the known effects of lead on biological systems are adverse (Chisolm 1977). Children are at particularly high risk for lead toxicity. They absorb ingested lead more efficiently than adults from the respiratory and gastrointestinal tracts and are slower to excrete lead (Hammond 1982).

Nutritional deficiencies in early childhood, especially the relatively common iron deficiency, can increase gastrointestinal lead absorption (Mahaffey 1982) at a time when the nervous system is most sensitive to insult.

In children, lead primarily affects red blood cell formation (as reflected in the elevation of erythrocyte protoporphyrin and resulting in anemia); the central and peripheral nervous system (leading to problems such as constipation, irritability, blindness, and encephalopathy); and the kidney. The severity of symptoms is thought to be related to the "dose" of lead to which a child is exposed. Over the years, the level of blood lead thought to be critical in distinguishing between toxicity and non-toxicity (the threshold level) has decreased as more sensitive tests of biologic, physiologic, and neurologic effects have been developed. In the 1950s and 1960s, levels above 60 micrograms/dl were considered abnormally high; currently, Centers for Disease Control guidelines define levels equal to or above 30 micrograms/dl as elevated (CDC 1978).

The morbidity attributable to chronic low level (asymptomatic) lead absorption (less than 30 micrograms/dl) is not well understood. Evidence is available for biological effects at blood lead levels below 30 micrograms/dl, although their clinical significance is not yet clear. Recent studies found evidence of changes in EEG brain wave patterns and CNS evoked potential responses in lead intoxicated children with relatively low blood lead levels (Otto et al. 1982; Otto et al. 1983). These changes persisted over the two years of follow-up. There is also evidence for adverse effects on biological functions including vitamin D metabolism at blood lead levels as low as 12 micrograms/dl (Rosen et al. 1981). Although the evidence is controversial, low levels of body lead are associated with subtle behavioral and neurologic deficits (Charney 1982b; Needleman et al. 1979; Rutter 1980). The serious nature of these effects combined with the high prevalence make lead toxicity a major health concern.

Children are exposed to lead via inhaled air and ingested food, water, leaded paint, dust, and soil. Lead is a heavy metal that is present throughout the natural and manmade environment (Landrigan 1982). Its concentration in air, water, and soil has increased dramatically since the Industrial Revolution, rising tenfold (from 10^5 to 10^6 tons per year over a 300-year period). A further increase (from 1 million to 3 million tons annually) occurred after the use of leaded fuels became commonplace 60 years ago (Settle and Patterson 1980, 1170). In 1981, auto emissions accounted for most (86 percent) of the generally nonrecoverable lead in the atmosphere with industry contributing the rest (Battye 1983).

The National Bureau of Standards (NBS) estimated that lead-based paint was used in 50 percent of housing built between 1940 and 1950 and in 5 percent of housing built between 1950 and 1960 (Gilsimm 1972). There is even evidence that some homes built in the 1970s contain leaded paint (NBS 1973) despite the existence of municipal ordinances from the 1950s and 1960s that prohibit its use. As a result, the 27 million homes built prior to

1940, a large proportion of the 22 million dwellings built between 1940 and 1960, and an unknown proportion built in the 1970s contain leaded paint (Bureau of the Census 1981).

Survey data also indicate that a significant proportion of houses contain peeling and chipping lead paint, which is particularly hazardous for young children (Shier and Hall 1977). On the other hand, approximately one third of the homes of affected children do not have lead paint hazards when inspected by local prevention program workers (CDC 1982a).

Dust is another important source of lead, especially in urban areas where lead from automobile exhaust is deposited on roadways, soil, and in dwellings in relatively large amounts. Lead-containing dust is an important contributor to subencephalopathic (low-level) lead poisoning (Charney 1982a).

Although the concentrations of lead in air, water, and food are thousands of times less than those found in paint, dust, and soil, they are generally thought to contribute to "background" levels in children, determining how much additional exposure is needed before toxicity occurs.

The Baltimore City Health Department was virtually the only city health department active in combating childhood lead poisoning before the 1950s (Lin-Fu 1982), so much of the information concerning medical and environmental interventions is based on studies in Baltimore.

Since the 1930s, several approaches using control of environmental sources and detection and treatment of exposed children have been developed to reduce the occurrence and sequelae of lead toxicity. Free blood lead testing services were first offered in 1935 for children suspected of having lead poisoning. Public health nurses investigated cases and educated parents in the 1940s. Cities passed ordinances to provide a legal base for lead paint removal from housing. Case finding combined with removal of lead paint from homes of affected children was the primary line of attack until the 1960s. The acute symptomatic cases diagnosed in Baltimore dropped from approximately 30 to 60 per year during the 1950s to half that number in 1967–70. The second approach used chelation therapy with calcium EDTA combined with dimercaprol to reduce the burden of lead in children hospitalized with acute toxicity. The introduction of this medical therapy contributed to a decline in deaths in Baltimore City (Chisolm 1968). Until 1963, the annual number of deaths ranged from 2 to 10; from then until 1970, there were only 4 deaths.

The third approach resulted from the development of a rapid and inexpensive analytical test for lead in paint in 1957 that enabled local health and housing authorities to launch a primary preventive program. For example, thousands of homes of children under three years of age who registered for care in one health district were visited for the purpose of identifying and enforcing correction of lead paint hazards before the children became poisoned. There has been opposition, however, to programs for removing leaded paint from housing because of the high costs of lead removal (Billick and Grey 1978), insufficient numbers of inspectors (Schucker et al. 1965), political conflict generated by placing economic demands on property owners and organized resistance of landlords (Clapp 1980), bureaucratic opposition to change (Bing 1980), and a widespread tendency to blame the victim's parents for negligent child supervision (Ryan 1971). A further obstacle to paint removal programs was the 1967 Supreme Court ruling (Camara v. the Municipal Court of San Francisco) that health inspections of homes during the day require a warrant.

Although deleading of homes contributed to reductions in deaths, paint removal itself can result in increases in body lead levels. Incomplete cleanup of paint chips and dust after abatement subjects children to new sources of readily ingestible lead. The burning and scraping technique and, to a lesser degree, the use of heat guns popular in some cities subject workers and children to concentrated levels of airborne lead and dust (Inskip 1984) leading to increased blood lead levels. Moreover, abatement practices are limited in scope and often deficient in work quality and safety. Intact paint that is not removed is subject to deterioration which leaves occupants at risk for further exposure (Tytun and Guinee 1972). One study found that 75 percent of a group of homes reduced of lead paint hazards one year earlier had new areas shedding leaded paint (New York City Health Dept. 1981).

In the 1970s, the Department of Housing and Urban Development financed the development and testing of new barrier materials and paint removal techniques for abating city dwellings (Billick and Grey 1978, appendices C, D) but this resulted in few if any new abatement regulations in cities with lead poisoning problems. The agency evaluated relative costs of various practices (Chapman 1976), but did not evaluate the effectiveness of the deleading strategies for reducing the blood lead levels of affected children.

More organized efforts to deal with lead poisoning were mounted in the late 1960s. At that time, local screening programs were initiated to identify asymptomatic children with undue lead absorption in order to prevent further exposure and progression to clinical toxicity (Lin-Fu 1982). Many reports documented the prevalence of elevated blood lead levels in children screened for the problem. Of high risk children screened in the late 1960s, 30–40 percent were found to have elevated lead levels. Evidence of a reduction in severity of cases found on screening began to appear in reports after early screening programs. Sachs (1974) reported that the number of children screened in Chicago increased each year from 1967 to 1971 and the proportion of children with blood lead concentrations over 50 micrograms/dl decreased from 8.5 percent to 2.3 percent. There was a similar drop in the proportion of preschool children with blood lead levels above 40 micrograms/dl (21–55 percent to 5–16 percent) and a significant decrease in the number of children who were symptomatic at the time of screening (12.2

percent to 4.2 percent). As these data were not population-based, they may reflect a real decline in the likelihood of acute toxicity and/or more intensive screening.

Cohen (1980) compared characteristics of children diagnosed and treated for lead poisoning at the Children's Hospital in Washington, D.C., during the early 1950s with those in the mid-1970s. In the 1970s, there were fewer children with central nervous system (CNS) symptoms or with markedly elevated blood lead levels (greater than 80 micrograms/dl).

A concerted attack on the problem at the federal level did not occur until the 1970s. During that decade, a variety of laws were passed and regulations promulgated. Mass screening programs to detect asymptomatic children with undue lead absorption were encouraged. The number of children screened in federally supported lead-based paint poisoning control projects has been reported by the CDC. From 1974 through 1978 approximately 400,000 children were screened each year. In the ensuing three years, the number screened increased progressively: 464,751, 502,925, and 535,730, respectively (CDC 1982c and quarterly reports). Concomitantly, the proportion of children categorized as Class II (mild elevation of blood lead) fell in the six years starting in October 1975 as follows: 5.8 percent, 5.0 percent, 4.4 percent, 4.7 percent, 3.5 percent, and 2.7 percent. The proportion of children categorized as Class III and Class IV (severe elevations of blood lead with concomitant evidence of biochemical toxicity) also fell: 2.7 percent, 2.5 percent, 2.1 percent, 2.3 percent, 1.8 percent, and 1.4 percent. However, the ratio of the number of more severely affected children (Class III and Class IV) to less severely affected children (Class II) has been increasing: 0.465, 0.491, 0.479, 0.500, 0.520, and 0.516, suggesting that although progression of symptoms to acute toxicity has been markedly decreased, the proportion of all children with undue lead absorption who are at highest priority for medical attention has not diminished and may be increasing (MMWR quarterly reports on Lead Poisoning Programs).

In 1978, the national Lead Paint Poisoning Prevention Program (consisting of approximately 60 local programs) was evaluated using a sample of 400 Class III children and 150 Class IV children chosen randomly from each geographic region. Based on several indicators, Kennedy (1978) concluded that most local programs were performing effectively. Over 90 percent of the children sampled began pediatric management, about three quarters of the homes of identified children were investigated (usually within two months), 80 percent of homes with lead paint hazards were reported to have been deleaded (with an average time lag of four months), and over 75 percent of the children showed some downward trend in blood lead and free erythroprotoporphyrin levels.

However, 58 and 85 percent of Class III and IV children, respectively, were lost to follow-up by one year. Moreover, the "success" rates of 75–80 percent meant that one fifth to one quarter of the children did not improve, have their homes inspected, or have identified lead hazards corrected or reduced. The data also revealed frequent long lag times before environmental follow-up and deleading. The proportion of children whose blood lead levels increased after initial detection varied directly with the length of time it took programs to provide follow-up medical and environmental services.

Despite these indications of benefit, local programs screen only 30 percent of the high-risk children nationwide and only 3 percent of all children under 6 years of age (National Research Council 1980, 93). Screening for lead poisoning has been included in the EPSDT program schedule of Medicaid, but this program has not reached a large proportion of eligible children as required. Also, although lead paint abatement requirements and practices developed decades ago reduced the occurrence of death or recurrent acute toxicity after a case had been detected, the continued use of these practices into the 1970s and 1980s has been ineffective in reducing the blood lead levels of children with low-level lead poisoning. Studies in Baltimore show no reduction in blood lead levels in either hospitalized children or nonhospitalized children with undue lead absorption one year after their homes were deleaded by current practices (Chisolm 1983; Charney et al. 1983). Children in Classes II and III commonly retain elevated levels for several years unless they return to housing free of lead paint. In 1980, approximately 25 percent of children hospitalized for lead chelation were readmitted within one year (John F. Kennedy Institute 1981). In 1982, 105 of 450 Class II and III children enrolled by one clinic were hospitalized; of these, 24 were being chelated for at least the third time (Chisolm, personal communication).

In contrast, lead poisoned children discharged from the hospital after chelation to lead-free public housing or totally renovated units do not develop rebounds in blood lead levels and they remain at low risk for further lead toxicity. Children who live in lead-free housing but frequently visit older dwellings tend to have higher blood lead levels than children who do not visit older dwellings (Chisolm 1983; John F. Kennedy Institute 1981).

The findings of a recently completed randomized controlled trial in Baltimore (Charney et al. 1983) showed that dust control combined with deleading for correcting paint hazards in homes resulted in an average 6.9 micrograms/dl reduction in blood lead levels in Class II children tested one year after abatement was performed, whereas deleading of paint alone resulted in no appreciable change.

Thus, although prevention based upon case-finding, screening, and removal of known sources of lead poisoning have undoubtedly been effective in reducing the occurrence of severe toxicity and death, evaluations have failed to provide unequivocal evidence of benefit of this approach to lead poisoning in its more chronic and insidious form.

Regulatory actions aimed at eliminating or reducing new inputs of lead into the environment, however, have had measurable success. For the country as a whole, the overall mean blood lead level concentration fell by 37 percent (15.8 to 10 micrograms/dl) between 1976 and 1980 (CDC 1982b). Decreases were found in all races and age groups. For children under 5 years of age the decline was just over 40 percent. The decline in mean blood lead levels increases the margin of safety of high-risk children before toxicity occurs.

These changes in blood lead levels parallel decreases in the production and use of leaded gasoline (CDC 1982b). Unleaded gas became generally available in 1975; between 1976 and 1980, lead used by refineries dropped by over 50 percent and nonmilitary sales of leaded gas dropped by about 30 percent. Between 1977 and 1980, mean ambient air lead concentrations in urban areas dropped by two-thirds (EPA 1978, 1979; National Filter Analysis Network 1982). The Environmental Protection Agency's standard for reducing the amount of lead in leaded gasoline took effect in 1980. By 1982, the amount of lead in gasoline was reduced by half (Chemical Week 1982).

By 1977, the lead content of all interior-use paint had been restricted to 0.06 percent by weight and prohibited in toys and furniture (Consumer Product Safety Commission 1977). The large existing reservoir of lead in dust and paint in and about the homes of urban children has not been specifically addressed by federal regulation, however, except for the small proportion of housing that is federally owned or assisted (Billick and Grey 1978).

The food industry removed sources of lead from infant milk and food products in the 1970s. The most important action was the elimination of soldered cans for infant formulas (Beloian and McDowell 1981). In the early 1980s, the Food and Drug Administration took steps to reduce lead in ceramic products (FDA 1979). These actions and a trend toward alternative packaging materials for foods in general may further reduce lead in food in the future.

These various environmental approaches to reducing the adverse effects of lead have undoubtedly been responsible for the recent decline in blood lead levels in the population. Continued reductions of lead in gasoline and food, which are primary contributors to background lead levels, and new methods of abatement and dust control could be expected to further increase the margin of safety resulting from the lower mean blood lead levels in the population. Despite the reductions of new inputs of lead in the environment, there remains a reservoir of lead in soil and existing house paint that will continue to be hazardous to many children and that will require persistent and improved efforts to screen high-risk populations, treat those who are affected, and remove sources of lead from their surroundings. Provenzano (1980) estimated the costs of lead-induced health and intellectual deficits in this country at $1 billion annually. Special education costs far exceed health care costs (69 versus 25 percent of total costs). At high-prevalence levels, such as those found in poor, urban black children, screening is cost-effective (Berwick and Komaroff 1982). Improved abatement procedures are required to break the cycle of chronic undue lead absorption in children identified as having elevated lead burdens. Better reporting systems are needed for assessing the impact of current and future interventions to deal with a persisting and pernicious health problem in childhood.

References

Battye B. Lead emission inventory, 1981 (Memo to John Haines). Environmental Protection Agency, Environmental Criteria and Assessment Office, Research Triangle Park, N.C., 1983.

Beloian A, McDowell M. Estimates of lead intake among children up to 5 years of age, 1973-1978 and 1980. Washington, D.C.: U.S. Food and Drug Administration, Bureau of Foods, Division of Nutrition, final internal report, 1981.

Berwick D, Komaroff A. Cost-effectiveness of lead screening. N Engl J Med 1982;306:1392-98.

Billick IH, Grey VE. Lead based paint poisoning research: review and evaluation, 1971-1977. Washington, D.C.: U.S. Dept. Housing and Urban Development, July 1978.

Bing S. The Massachusetts childhood lead poisoning prevention program: an advocate's view. In: Needleman HL. Low level lead exposure: the implications of current research. New York: Raven Press, 1980:293-97.

Bureau of the Census. Statistical abstracts of the United States 1980, 101st ed. Washington, D.C.: U.S. Dept. of Commerce, 1981.

Camara v. Municipal Court of the City and County of San Francisco, 387 U.S. 523 (1967).

CDC (Centers for Disease Control). Preventing lead poisoning in young children: a statement by the CDC. Washington, D.C.: U.S. Dept. HEW, PHS, April 1978.

CDC (Centers for Disease Control). Surveillance of childhood lead poisoning. MMWR March 12, 1982a;31(9):118-19.

CDC (Centers for Disease Control). Surveillance of childhood lead poisoning. MMWR March 19, 1982b;31(10):132-34.

CDC (Centers for Disease Control). Annual summary 1981. MMWR October 1982c;30(54):112-13.

Chapman RE. Economic analysis of experimental lead paint abatement methods: phase I. Washington, D.C.: National Bureau of Standards technical note 922, 1976.

Charney E. Lead poisoning in children: the case against household lead dust. In: Chisolm, O'Hara, eds., op. cit., 1982a:79-88.

Charney E. Sub-encephalopathic lead poisoning: central nervous system effects in children. In: Chisolm, O'Hara, eds., op. cit., 1982b:35-42.

Charney E, Kessler B, Farfel M, Jackson D. Childhood lead poisoning: a controlled trial of the effect of dust-control measures on blood lead levels. N Engl J Med 1983;309(18):1089-93.

Chemical Week. EPA Lightens up on Anti-Knocks. April 14, 1982;130:13.

Chisolm JJ. The use of chelating agents in the treatment of acute and chronic lead intoxication in childhood. J Pediatr 1968;73:1-38.

Chisolm JJ. Lead poisoning. In: Rudolph AM, ed. Pediatrics, 16th ed. New York: Appleton-Century-Crofts, 1977:797-806.

Chisolm JJ. Relationship between level of lead absorption in children and type, age and condition of housing in Baltimore, Maryland, U.S.A., 1983. Paper presented at the Conference on Heavy Metals in the Environment. Weidelberg, West Germany. Sept. 1983 CEP Consultants. Edinburgh.

Chisolm JJ, O'Hara DM, eds. Lead absorption in children: management, clinical and environmental aspects. Baltimore: Urban & Schwarzenberg, 1982.

Clapp R. The Massachusetts childhood lead poisoning prevention program. In: Needleman L. Low level lead exposure: the implications of current research. New York: Raven Press, 1980:285-91.

Cohen GJ. Lead poisoning: 20 years later. Clin Pediatr 1980;19:245-50.

Consumer Product Safety Commission. Lead-containing paint and certain consumer products bearing lead containing paint, 16 CFR 1303 federal register: 44192-44202, Sept. 1, 1977.

EPA (Environmental Protection Agency). Air quality data for metals, 1975. In: The national air surveillance network, Research Triangle Park, N.C.: Office of Research and Development, 1978. EPA report no. (EPA) 600/4-78-059.

EPA (Environmental Protection Agency). Air quality data for metals, 1976. In: The national air surveillance network, Research Triangle Park, N.C.: Office of Research and Development, 1979. EPA report no. (EPA) 600/4-79-054.

FDA (Food and Drug Administration) Administrative guideline 7417.00 pottery (ceramics)-lead contamination. 1979.

Gilsimm J. Estimate of the nature and extent of lead paint poisoning in the United States. Washington, D.C.: National Bureau of Standards, 1972. Technical note 746.

Hammond P. Metabolism of lead. In: Chisolm, O'Hara, eds., op. cit., 1982:11-20.

Inskip MJ. Lead-based paints: potential hazards associated with their presence and removal. In: London Environmental Supplement to the London Environmental Bulletin 1984;6:1-7.

John F. Kennedy Institute for Handicapped Children. Report to the mayor: lead poisoning prevention in Baltimore City in the 1980s. January 1, 1981.

Kennedy FD. The childhood lead poisoning prevention program: an evalua-

tion. Unpublished study submitted to the Center for Disease Control, U.S. Public Health Service, 1978.
Landrigan PJ. Epidemiology of lead and other metal poisonings in children. In: Finberg L, Miller RW, eds. Chemical and radiation hazards to children. Columbus, Ohio: Ross Laboratories, 1982:40-49.
Levinson A, Harris LH. Lead encephalopathy in children. J Pediatr 1936;8:2-15.
Lin-Fu J. The evolution of childhood lead poisoning as a public health problem. In: Chisolm, O'Hara, eds., op. cit., 1982:1-10.
Mahaffey KR. Role of nutrition in prevention of pediatric lead toxicity. In: Chisolm, O'Hara, eds., op. cit., 1982:63-78.
Mahaffey KR, Annest JL, Roberts J, Murphy RS. National estimates of blood lead levels: United States, 1976-1980—association with selected demographic and socioeconomic factors. N Engl J Med 1982;307:573-79.
NBS (National Bureau of Standards). Lead paint survey sampling plan and preliminary screening. Washington, D.C., 1973, report 10958.
National Filter Analysis Network. Environmental monitoring systems. Research Triangle Park, N.C.: U.S. Environmental Protection Agency, 1982.
National Research Council. Lead in the human environment: a report prepared by the committee on lead in the human environment. Washington, D.C.: National Academy of Sciences Press, 1980.
Needleman HL, Gunnoe C, Leviton A, et al. Deficits in psychologic and classroom performance of children with elevated dentine lead levels. N Engl J Med 1979;300(13):689-95.
New York City Health Department. The evaluation of alternative intervention and hazard abatement techniques for the control of childhood lead based paint poisoning. Draft Final Report, Submitted to Dept. HUD, Environment Hazard Research Div., Sept. 1981.
Otto D, Benignus V, Muller K, et al. Effects of low to moderate lead exposure on slow cortical potentials in young children: two year follow-up study. Neurobehav Toxicol Teratol 1982;4:733-37.
Otto D, Benignus V, Muller K, Barton C. Electrophysiologic evidence of changes in CNS function at low to moderate blood lead levels in children. In: Rutter M, Jones RR, eds. Lead versus health: source and effects of low level lead exposure. New York: John Wiley & Sons, 1983:319-31.
Provenzano G. The social costs of excessive lead exposure during childhood. In: Needleman HL. Low level lead exposure: the implications of current research. New York: Raven Press, 1980:299-315.
Rosen JF, Chesney RW, Hamstra A, DeLuca HF, Mahaffey KR. Reduction in 1,25 dihydroxy vitamin D in children with increased lead absorption. In: Brown S, David D., eds. Organ-directed toxicity: chemical indices and mechanisms. New York: Pergamon Press, 1981:91-95.

Rutter M. Raised lead levels and impaired cognitive/behavioral functioning: a review of the evidence. Dev Med Child Neurol (suppl) 1980;22:1–26.

Ryan W. Blaming the victim. New York: Vantage Press, 1971.

Sachs H. Effect of a screening program in changing patterns of lead poisoning. Environ Health Perspect 1974;7:41–45.

Schucker GW, Edward H, Vail EH, Kelly EB, Kaplan E. Prevention of lead paint poisoning among Baltimore children—a hard sell program. Public Health Rep 1965;80:969–74.

Settle DM, Patterson CC. Lead in albacore: guide to lead pollution in Americans. Science 1980;207:1167–76.

Shier DR, Hall W. Analysis of housing data collected in a lead-based paint survey in Pittsburgh, Pennsylvania, part I. Washington, D.C.: National Bureau of Standards, 1977. interagency report 77–1250.

Thomas HM, Blackfan KD. Recurrent meningitis due to lead in a child of five years. Am J Dis Child 1914;8:337–80.

Tytun A, Guinee VF. X-2 housing survey. New York City Health Department report, March 23, 1972.

11
Iron-Deficiency Anemia

Nancy Hutton and Barbara Starfield

Iron-deficiency anemia is the most common hematologic disorder as well as the most common expression of nutritional deficiency in children. Infants and young children are especially prone to this problem because their rapid physical growth depletes body iron stores at an age when their diet often contains insufficient iron for growth requirements. Anemia due to iron deficiency affects many organ systems, causing numerous symptoms (Lanzkowsky 1978; Smith and Rios 1974). Fatigue, weakness, irritability, inability to concentrate, anorexia, pica, and acute gastrointestinal blood loss are not uncommon in anemic children. Severe anemia may result in exudative enteropathy, malabsorption, and cardiovascular compromise. Recently, the iron deficient state rather than the anemic state has been implicated in behavioral changes in children, particularly irritability and inattention (Oski and Stockman 1980). These symptoms disappear shortly after the institution of iron therapy, prior to a change in circulatory hemoglobin. The efficacy of iron in preventing and treating iron deficiency anemia has been documented (Starfield 1977). It can be prevented by beginning an iron-fortified diet early in infancy (Marsh et al. 1959).

Several studies have been conducted since 1930 to document the prevalence of anemia in young children of varying age, race, and socioeconomic status (Table 4). These studies cannot be strictly compared due to differences in population selection and laboratory techniques, but the higher prevalence of anemia among blacks and children of lower socioeconomic status is consistent. The prevalence seems to have decreased in the 1970s.

Guest and Brown (1957) presented hematologic data selected at random from white children seen in the hospital, outpatient clinics, and orphanages between 1932 and 1942 in Cincinnati. These children were of varying economic backgrounds and had no primary blood dyscrasia. One fifth (20.1 percent) of the children aged 6 months to 3 years had hemoglobin concentrations less than 10.5 grams/dl. Of the 295 children between the ages of 12 and 24 months, 26.4 percent had levels below 10.5 grams/dl. The authors also

Table 4
Summary of Studies Reporting Prevalence of Iron-Deficiency Anemia in Young Children (6 months–5 years), 1932–74

Study Location and Authors	Study Dates	Race	Socioeconomic Status	Age	Percentage of Children with Low Hemoglobin Concentration		
					<10.0 gm/dl	<10.5 gm/dl	<11.0 gm/dl
Cincinnati, OH (Guest and Brown 1957)	1932–42	white	unknown	6–36 mos.		20	
				12–24 mos.		26.4	
	1954	white	unknown	6–36 mos.		22	
				12–24 mos.		30	
Washington, D.C. (Gutelius 1969)	1965	black	low income	6–36 mos.	40		
				12–23 mos.	48		
Panorama City, CA (Fuerth 1971)	1959	white	middle income	12 mos.	6.3		21.6
	1969	white	middle income	9 mos.	3		14
National sample (Owen et al. 1970, 1971, 1973)	1969–70	all	lowest SES rank	12–23 mos.	14		27
		all	upper middle SES rank	12–23 mos.	0		3
National sample (NCHS 1974, 1982)	1971–72	white	below poverty level	1–5 yrs.	5		
		white	above poverty level	1–5 yrs.	1.2		
		black	below poverty level	1–5 yrs.	9.3		
		black	above poverty level	1–5 yrs.	7.7		
	1971–74	white males	all	12–24 mos.			14.9
		black males	all	12–24 mos.			42.1
		white females	all	12–24 mos.			10.5
		black females	all	12–24 mos.			21.8

reported Lahey's findings in 314 children between the ages of 6 months and 3 years admitted successively to Cincinnati Children's Hospital in 1954; 22 percent of these children had hemoglobins less than 10.5 grams/dl. Of 140 children between 12 and 24 months, 30 percent fell below this level. Because children with other hematologic and systemic diseases causing anemia were excluded from study in both groups, the authors concluded that these were good approximations of the prevalence of iron deficiency anemia in white children of Cincinnati and that these rates were unchanged during the 1930s and 1940s.

Gutelius (1969) reported hemoglobin and hematocrit levels in low-income black children in Washington, D.C., during 1965 when routine screening was initiated. Preschool children over age 2 months seen at the Child Health Center of the Children's Hospital who had no previous hemoglobin determination recorded were included in the report. Iron deficiency anemia was defined as a hemoglobin less than 10.0 grams/dl with evidence of microcytosis and hypochromia on blood smear. Two out of five (39.5 percent) of 299 children between 6 months and 3 years of age fell into this category. At ages 12–23 months, 48.3 percent were found to have anemia.

Fuerth (1971) compared the incidence of anemia in white, middle-class infants belonging to the Kaiser Health Plan in Panorama City, California, during 1959 and 1969. During 1959, 21.6 percent of 526 children tested at 1 year of age had hemoglobin concentrations less than 11.0 grams/dl; 6.3 percent of this surveyed group had hemoglobins less than 10.0 grams/dl. During 1969, 315 children were tested at 9 months of age; 14 percent of these had hemoglobins less than 11.0 grams/dl and 3 percent were below 10.0 grams/dl. These data show a decrease in incidence of low hemoglobin over the decade of the 1960s when nutritional and screening recommendations were being implemented. The percentages of children with low values were consistently lower, in both periods, than those reported in low socioeconomic population groups.

In a series of articles, Owen et al. (1970, 1971, 1973) reported results of a national nutritional survey carried out during 1969–70 on a cross-sectional sample of the preschool population between 12 and 71 months of age. These investigators listed mean values for hemoglobin, hematocrit, and iron by age and socioeconomic status, and they compared the data by race when socioeconomic status was comparable. In 12–23 month olds, 27 percent had hemoglobin values below 11.0 grams/dl and 14 percent were below 10.0 grams/dl within the lowest SES rank. In contrast, children of the same age, but in the upper middle stratum, were much less likely to be anemic. Only 3 percent were below 11.0 grams/dl of hemoglobin and none were below 10.0 grams/dl.

Preliminary data from the first National Health and Nutritional Examination Survey (NCHS 1974) conducted during 1971–72 revealed that approximately 5 percent of white children ages 1–5 years whose families fell below the poverty level had a hemoglobin concentration less than 10.0 grams/dl.

Only 1.2 percent of white children in this age group above the poverty level were this anemic. In both income groups, there were higher percentages of black children in this age group with low hemoglobins compared with white children. Almost 8 percent (7.7 percent) of black children above the poverty level and 9.3 percent of those below the poverty level had hemoglobins below 10.0 grams/dl. Transferrin saturation less than 15 percent, a biochemical indicator for iron deficiency, was found in 14 percent of 1–5 year olds below the poverty level in contrast to less than 10 percent of 1–5 year olds above the poverty level. When transferrin saturation levels were determined within racial groups, white children below the poverty level had a higher rate than those above the poverty level (12.9 percent versus 8.6 percent), but black children showed the reverse (below poverty level: 15.8 percent; above poverty level: 22.1 percent). When the prevalence was determined by age group, peak rates were found at 12–24 months in all groups (NCHS 1982). Among black 1 year olds, 42.1 percent of boys and 21.8 percent of girls had hemoglobin levels less than 11.0 grams/dl. This decreased to a nadir of 6.4 percent and 2.8 percent who were anemic at 4 and 5 years of age, respectively. In white children, these rates were 14.9 percent of boys decreasing to 0.9 percent and 10.5 percent of girls decreasing to 1.7 percent between the ages of 1 and 5 years.

The above studies seem to indicate a racial difference in hematologic parameters. Possible explanations for this phenomenon are that socioeconomic status is at least in part confounding the comparisons, that hemoglobin concentrations are lower in blacks due to a high incidence of genetic hemoglobinopathies (Pearson et al. 1967), or that the normal distribution is shifted to a different mean for some unknown reason (Owen et al. 1973). Dallman et al. (1967) studied 2,774 children ages 5–14 years enrolled at Kaiser-Permanente in San Francisco during 1973–75. The racial mixture of the group was 62 percent white, 27 percent black, and 11 percent oriental; the SES of all children was comparable. After excluding children with microcytosis, abnormal hemoglobin electrophoresis, and abnormal G6PD screen, blacks had median hemoglobin values 0.5 grams/dl less than whites or orientals. (Preschool children were not studied.) Although this study lends support to the theory that blacks and whites differ in the mean and distribution of normal hemoglobin values, it indicates that the difference is quite small. Racial differences alone could not explain the impressive findings of extent of anemia in low socioeconomic black children in studies conducted in 1965–66 by Gutelius (1969) or those of Andelman and Sered (1966) (see below) in 1965–66.

Iron supplementation is efficacious in the prevention of iron-deficiency anemia. The effect of iron-fortified diets or iron supplementation on the hemoglobin levels in normal infants was studied between 1956 and 1970. During 1956–57, Marsh et al. (1959) followed infants for the first 9 months of life in groups according to birth weight (premature or full term). They compared three feeding regimens (commercial infant formula with or without iron fortification, and evaporated milk formula) and found that hemoglobin, hematocrit, and serum iron were higher in the iron-fortified group after 3 months of age. This difference persisted throughout the remainder of the 9 months.

In 1966, Andelman and Sered reported a study of 1,048 infants from the lowest socioeconomic district in Chicago who were randomly selected and assigned to a control group and a study group. Control group infants (445) were fed infant formula without iron supplementation and infants in the study group (603) were fed formula containing 12 mgm elemental iron per quart. The population in each group was almost entirely nonwhite and the groups were similar in living conditions, family size, birth weight, sex, and maternal age and parity. Children were observed at routine visits for well child care until age 18 months and blood studies were performed at each visit. Mean hemoglobin concentration for 1 to 1½ year olds in the control group were 10.4–10.6 grams/dl. The study group's mean for this age group was 11.7–11.6 grams/dl, a substantially different result. Three quarters (76 percent) of the control group developed iron-deficiency anemia, most before the age of 12 months, in contrast to 9 percent of the study group. More than half the latter group did not become anemic until 6–12 months after discontinuing iron supplementation.

Brigety and Pearson (1970) reported that short-term dietary supplementation in low-socioeconomic, black, preschool children in 1970 was followed by an increase in hematocrit of at least 2 percent in 14 percent of this group. This increased the mean value of hematocrits by a small but statistically significant amount. A second group of children from the same preschool programs received the same diet as well as 30 mgm of elemental iron supplementation per school day and showed an even greater increase in the mean and distribution of hematocrits. An increase of at least 2 percent was detected in 33 percent of the children in this second group. Burman (1972) reported higher hemoglobin levels in boys under age 24 months from low socioeconomic strata in England whose diets were supplemented with iron when compared with a similar group receiving placebo.

Based on evidence of high prevalence of anemia, particularly during the second year of life and in children from low socioeconomic groups, and the availability of a simple method for prevention, the American Academy of Pediatrics published recommendations for meeting the iron requirements of infants in 1969 (American Academy of Pediatrics 1969). These were updated in 1971 and 1976 (American Academy of Pediatrics 1971, 1976). Breast milk or iron fortified infant formula was recommended until at least age 12 months. The WIC program, a supplemental food program for pregnant or lactating women, infants, and children was authorized in 1972. The Academy recommended screening for anemia between ages 9 and 12 months in term infants and between 6 and 9 months in low birth weight infants (American Academy of Pediatrics 1976). Access to early diagnosis and treatment for children from low socioeconomic strata increased with

Medicaid support, including the EPSDT program, which was finally implemented for infants and children under age 6 in February, 1972 and for all children under 21 years by July, 1973.

To evaluate the effectiveness of the WIC program, health measures for 41,330 children from 14 states participating in the program during 1974–76 were studied (Edozien et al. 1979). Comparisons were made between children of similar ages who were about to enroll in WIC and those who had participated for 6 months and for 11 months. The possibility of using each child as his own control was considered, but the effects of aging were felt to confound this sort of comparison. One third (33 percent) of the children who enrolled in the program between 12 and 23 months of age had hemoglobin values less than 11.0 grams/dl at the initial measurement. Half of these children had a transferrin saturation less than 15 percent. Anemia rates were highest among blacks and American Indians. Within age groups, there was a significant reduction in the prevalence of anemia between children seen initially and children of the same age in the program for six months. This reduction in anemia continued to the 11-month visit within the 12–23 month age groups. Also, the distribution of hemoglobin values in all children 12–47 months old shifted to higher mean and median values after six months in the program as compared with children of similar age just enrolling in the program.

Rush (1982) reported the results of an unpublished study of several smaller evaluations of the effect of the WIC program. The investigators (Graham and Greenberg) concluded that benefits may have occurred but that they may have been due to participation in general health programs or to other factors uncontrolled by the research design rather than to the WIC program.

In a more recent study in sibling pairs of the cognitive effects of nutritional supplementation by the WIC program (Hicks et al. 1982), significantly higher scores on multiple tests of cognitive function were found in children who had been supplemented from an earlier age and for a longer period of time. Health measures including height for age, weight for height, presence of anemia, and school absences were obtained from public health clinic records and were also studied. Although performance was better in the group supplemented at an early age, the differences reached statistical significance only for height appropriate for age. Although anemia (hemoglobin less than 11 or hematocrit less than 34) was noted at 17.4 percent of clinic visits by children in the late supplementation group and 14.2 percent of visits by the early group, this difference did not reach statistical significance. This study has been regarded as "an important first step" in evaluating the benefits of WIC participation and a challenge to further investigators (Rush 1982).

In a study conducted in Baltimore, Starfield and Scheff showed that anemic children were more likely to be found to have normal hematologic values six months later if the medical facility had made the family aware of the anemia, although iron therapy itself was an important predictor of improvement if the family was not aware of the reason for it. That is, access to medical care and resulting recognition or diagnosis of the problem resulted in improvement as compared with children in whom the anemia was not recognized (Starfield 1977).

In summary, the incidence and prevalence studies done in the past define a population of children at risk: those less than 3 years of age, especially during the second year of life, and those of low socioeconomic status. Prevention of iron deficiency anemia is straightforward. No studies have determined whether or not the prevalence of iron deficiency anemia is changing over time in the population as a whole or in particular subpopulations, although the overwhelming clinical impression is that anemia is less common, especially severe anemia due to iron deficiency. Intervention, whether on an individual or a program basis, seems to reduce the frequency of anemia both by preventing it and detecting it in its early stages.

References

Andelman M, Sered B. Utilization of dietary iron by term infants. Am J Dis Child 1966;111:45–55.

American Academy of Pediatrics, Committee on Nutrition. Iron balance and requirements in infancy. Pediatrics 1969;43:134–42.

American Academy of Pediatrics, Committee on Nutrition. Iron-fortified formulas. Pediatrics 1971;47:786.

American Academy of Pediatrics, Committee on Nutrition. Iron supplementation for infants. Pediatrics 1976;58:765–67.

Brigety R, Pearson H. Effects of dietary and iron supplementation on hematocrit levels in preschool children. J Pediatr 1970;76:757–60.

Burman D. Haemoglobin levels in normal infants aged 3 to 24 months, and the effect of iron. Arch Dis Child 1972;47:261–71.

Dallman P, Barr G, Allen C, et al. Anemia in preschool children in the United States of America. Pediatr Res 1967;1:169–72.

Edozien J, Switzer B, Bryan R. Medical evaluation of the special supplemental food program for women, infants, and children. Am J Clin Nutr 1979;32:677–92.

Fuerth J. Incidence of anemia in full-term infants seen in private practice. J Pediatr 1971;79:560–62.

Guest G, Brown E. Erythrocytes and hemoglobin of the blood in infancy and childhood. Am J Dis Child 1957;93:486–509.

Gutelius M. The problem of iron deficiency anemia in preschool Negro children. Am J Public Health 1969;59:290–95.

Hicks L, Langham R, Takenaka J. Cognitive and health measures following early nutritional supplementation: a sibling study. Am J Public Health 1982;72:1110–18.

Lanzkowsky P. Iron metabolism and iron deficiency anemia. In: Miller DR, Pearson HA, Smith CH. eds. Smith's blood diseases in infancy and childhood, 4th ed. St. Louis: Mosby, 1978:173-211.

Marsh A, Long H, Stierwart E. Comparative hematologic response to iron fortification of a milk formula for infants. Pediatrics 1959;24:404-12.

NCHS (National Center for Health Statistics). Preliminary findings of the first health and nutrition examination survey, United States 1971-1972: dietary intake and biochemical findings, 1974. Washington, D.C.: U.S. Government Printing Office, 1974 (DHEW publication no. (HRA)74-1219).

NCHS (National Center for Health Statistics). Diet and iron status, a study of relationships: United States, 1971-1974. Vital Health Stat, series 11, no. 229, 1982.

Oski F, Stockman J. Anemia due to inadequate iron sources or poor iron utilization. Pediatr Clin North Am 1980;27:237-52.

Owen G, Lubin A, Garry P. Preschool children in the United States: who has iron deficiency? J Pediatr 1971;79:563-68.

Owen G, Lubin A, Garry P. Hemoglobin levels according to age, race and transferrin saturation in preschool children of comparable socioeconomic status. J Pediatr 1973;82:850-51.

Owen G, Nelson C, Garry P. Nutritional status of preschool children: hemoglobin, hematocrit, and plasma iron values. J Pediatr 1970;76:761-63.

Pearson H, Abrams I. Fernbach D, et al. Anemia in preschool children in the United States of America. Pediatr Res 1967;1:169-72.

Rush D. Is WIC worthwhile? editorial commentary. Am J Public Health 1982;72:1101-3.

Smith N, Rios E. Iron metabolism and iron deficiency in infancy and childhood. Adv Pediatr 1974;21:239-80.

Starfield B. Iron-deficiency anemia. In: Harvard Child Health Project. Children's medical care needs and treatments. Cambridge, Mass.: Ballinger, 1977:77-120.

Part III

Child Health Problems Amenable to Treatment by Medical Care through Prevention of Complications or Sequelae

12
Diabetes: Prevention of Ketoacidosis

Barbara Starfield

Diabetes is not rare in childhood. The estimated prevalence is about 2 per 1,000 population under age 20 and 1.6 per 1,000 at ages 0–16 (NDDG 1980). Diabetes has been reported as slightly less prevalent among poor children than among nonpoor children (NDDG 1980; Colle et al. 1981), although recent data suggest that the social class relationship has disappeared (La Porte et al. 1981). As the prevalence of diabetes is much higher among poor adults than among nonpoor adults, the earlier lower prevalence rates among poor children suggests previous underdiagnosis in poor populations.

The incidence and prevalence of diabetes rose considerably between 1946 and 1979 (NDDG 1980; Sultz et al. 1972), with an accelerated rate of increase after 1965 (NDDG 1980; North et al. 1977). (In adults, the acceleration in rate of increased diagnosis antedated 1965.) In 1946 the annual incidence rate was 9.9 per 100,000 for children under age 15 (Sultz et al. 1972); between 1947 and 1951 the annual incidence rate was no higher than 7.5 per 100,000. By 1958 the rate had risen to about 12.5 per 100,000 where it remained (NDDG 1980; Fishbein et al. 1982). Rates of diabetes vary considerably with age, even in childhood. In 1979–80, the annual incidence rates (per 100,000 children at risk) were 6 at ages 0–4, 13 at ages 5–9, 19 at ages 10–14, and 11 at ages 15–19 (Fishbein et al. 1982). The increases between 1946 and 1979 were not due to a changing age distribution of the population (Sultz et al. 1972; North et al. 1977) but rather were likely to have been due at least in part to greater access to care and recognition of the condition. For example, from 1949 to 1961, rates of incidence among nonwhite children increased relatively more than among whites (Sultz et al. 1972), suggesting that the diagnosis of those who had been relatively deprived of access to medical care earlier in the period may have been missed, possibly with deaths unattributed to diabetes.

Children who are of low socioeconomic status (SES) are at greater risk of dying, even if their diabetes is known. In a community study of children during the period from 1949 to 1961, the case fatality for children 0–15 was 3.1 percent for low SES children, 1.4 percent for middle SES children, and 1.3 percent for high SES children; mortality rates per 1,000 patient years of diabetes were 7.2, 3.1, and 3.0, respectively (Sultz et al. 1972).

Diabetic ketoacidosis (DKA) is a much more common complication in children than in adults (Faich et al. 1983). In 1979–80, the annual rate of its occurrence was 533 per 10,000 diabetics under age 15, as compared with rates of 109 at ages 15–44, 21 at ages 45–64, and 28 at ages above 64. Without rapid hospitalization and care for ketoacidosis, death may result even before the diagnosis is made if it is the first episode.

Although more recent data on rates of hospitalization among diabetics are not available, 13 percent of diabetic children (under age 15) were hospitalized each year from 1949 to 1961 (Sultz et al. 1972). Among diabetic patients under age 20, 60 percent of all hospital admissions primarily for diabetes are a result of ketoacidosis and over one third of all admissions of diabetics are for ketoacidosis (NDDG 1980; Sultz et al. 1972). Inferences from other data suggest that approximately the same or perhaps a slightly higher proportion of diabetics are hospitalized today as in 1949–61. (For example, in 1979–80 the rate of hospitalization for diabetic ketoacidosis was 533 per 10,000 diabetics per year. If the proportion of diabetic hospitalizations that were for DKA was 30 percent, then the rate of hospitalization among diabetics was 1,777 per 10,000 or 17.8 percent.)

Evidence of inadequate control of diabetes among poor children is suggested by data on rehospitalizations and case fatality, both of which are higher among poor children. Among children hospitalized for newly diagnosed diabetes, 71 percent of insulin-dependent diabetics under age 30 who were living in poverty (according to census tract of residence) were readmitted during a two-year period. In contrast, only 17 percent of patients categorized as of high SES, 25 percent of middle SES patients, and 15 percent of low SES patients were readmitted in the same time period. For previously known diabetics, 40 percent of high SES, 50 percent of middle SES, 62 percent of low SES, and 73 percent of individuals in poverty had readmissions in the two years (Fishbein and Faich 1982).

The importance of a mechanism for financing care for diabetics is indicated by the impact on families of the considerable cost of management of the illness and its complications. In 1976, the average length of stay in the hospital for diabetics under age 17 was 5.5 days (NDDG 1980). In the year most costly to families of diabetic children (from 1946 to 1961) in Erie County, New York, 85 percent of hospitalization costs, 38 percent of physician costs, and less than 2 percent of costs for medication were covered by insurance; out-of-pocket costs for noninsured care were 37 percent of the total cost and were evenly divided among hospital care, physician care, and medication. Almost two-thirds of maintenance costs, calculated in 1963, were paid out of pocket. In fact, the mean costs of medication and "other" expenses were higher than all out-of-pocket costs in the costliest year. They consumed 3.4 percent of gross family income and 12 of 33 families (36 percent) spent between 6 percent and 15 percent of their gross income on these costs.

Of all diabetics under age 30 hospitalized in Rhode Island in a three year period (1979–81), 57 percent were covered by Blue Cross/Blue Shield, 23 percent by Medicaid, 4 percent by personal cash, and 16 percent by other (including HMO, commercial insurance, public programs, and unknown) (Fishbein and Faich 1982).

In contrast to the relatively sparse data on long-term benefits of therapy for the prevention of the complications of diabetes, there is substantial theoretical basis for benefit of medical care and actual demonstration of its usefulness in preventing ketoacidosis.

Individuals with diabetic ketoacidosis have mean blood insulin levels that are not substantially different from normal subjects after an overnight fast (Schade and Eaton 1979). However, diabetics are unable to raise their blood insulin levels to concentrations attained by normal subjects in response to stress of a variety of types. Maintenance therapy with insulin does not enable such individuals to deal with stress imposed by infection, fasting, or fever. Stress in the form of infection is a much more common (56 percent) precipitating cause of ketoacidosis than is insulin withdrawal (Hochaday and Alberti, cited in Schade and Eaton 1979); diabetics secrete excess stress hormones in response to stress and these hormones are themselves implicated in the pathogenesis of DKA. Thus, critical to the prevention and early management of DKA is access to medical care.

Reduction in stress responses by the use of antibiotics to treat infection and the elimination of fever and dehydration (which also facilitate the development of ketoacidosis) are the mechanisms by which medical care would be expected to reduce the need for hospitalization for DKA and to reduce case fatality.

A study of deaths from diabetes for the years 1968 to 1979 in the state of Washington indicated that 29 percent of all deaths due to acute diabetic complications occurred at home or en route to the hospital, suggesting either problems with access to care, problems with disease self-management, psychosocial difficulties, or poor advice from providers (Connell and Louden 1983).

Documentation of the beneficial impact of increased access to care has been provided by several investigations. All were studies in which experiences before an intervention were compared with those after the intervention. Although none were randomized controlled trials, the consistency of findings of studies done in diverse locales and at different times during the 1970s suggest that their findings are valid and generalizable. (Note: There are a number of evaluations of demonstration projects to educate individuals with diabetes. Since these programs are not widespread, and they do not deal with issues of access to care as commonly delivered, they are not included in this review.)

Miller and Goldstein (1972) surveyed admissions (presumably all adults) to the Los Angeles County University of Southern California Medical Center for a five-year period ending in 1967 and found that as many as 50 percent of admissions could have been prevented if medical care had been readily available to those patients. The system in existence (regular scheduled follow-up, visits to emergency room for sporadic care) made it difficult for patients to obtain help from an individual or facility that was familiar with them and led to poor management, drug duplications, and unnecessary admissions of individuals who could have been treated as outpatients. Patients who elected to wait for their regularly scheduled visit rather than seek needed care often had to be admitted with an urgent problem. In 1969 access to care for advice or prescription refills was made available 24 hours a day, seven days a week; patients appearing in the emergency room were referred to the telephone answering service unless they appeared with trauma. Although the total diabetic population increased from 4,000 to 6,000 from 1968 to 1970, the number of admissions decreased from 2,680 to 1,250 despite the aging of the population, with cost savings on the order of $3 million. The occurrence of diabetic coma was reduced from 300 to less than 100 in the same period.

Runyan et al. (1980) conducted an analysis of seven years of experience after instituting a decentralized network of neighborhood health clinics and 20 satellite clinics staffed by nurses in 1963 in Memphis. This analysis of the experiences of a sample of adult patients who survived over the seven-year period indicated that the hospitalization rate in the seventh year was 155 days per 1,000 patients compared with 4,809 days in the year before the program. For the entire seven years the mean yearly hospitalization rate was 2,282 days per 1,000 patients, or 47 percent of the figure prior to the programs. For DKA, the decrease was 69 percent. During this period, the annual rate of ambulatory visits to the decentralized facilities remained constant beginning with the third year of observation, and exceeded the preprogram rate by 9 percent.

The study of diabetic adults conducted by Davidson and colleagues from 1971 to 1978 indicated that increased access to care that emphasized intensive nutritional control and discontinuance of oral hypoglycemic agents led to a reduction in the prevalence of DKA by 143 percent although the report does not indicate over what period of time this occurred or after what time period subsequent to the intervention (Davidson et al. 1979).

Giordano et al. (1977) studied the impact of increased access to care, provided by a nurse specialist and a physician sharing 24-hour, on-call responsibility, by measuring changes in hospital days of diabetic children. In this program access was available to all patients, families, practicing physicians, and other health professionals in north-central Florida. As compared with preprogram experiences, the vast majority (86 percent) of hospital days for newly diagnosed patients were prevented; over 60 percent of hospital days for established cases (61 percent for the first program year, 81 percent for the second program year) were prevented. Although the base population is not well described in this study, making it difficult to interpret the overall significance of these changes, it is apparent that substantial reductions in the need for hospitalization occurred.

Hoffman et al. (1978) analyzed data on hospitalizations before and after institution in 1974 of a program to provide telephone access to 160 children and adolescents (ages 1 month to 17 years) enrolled at the Children's Hospital of Michigan. The telephone access was designed to provide advice about illness (92 percent of calls), to facilitate access to care for acute conditions (2 percent of calls), to answer specific questions (5 percent), and to facilitate prescription refills (1 percent). The average number of admissions per year per individual dropped from 0.60 and 0.69 in 1972–73 and 1973–74 to 0.56 in 1974–75, 0.09 in 1975–76, and 0.05 in 1976–77. There were no repeat admissions in the three years after telephone access was instituted.

On the basis of the changing epidemiology of diabetes, evidence of its greater seriousness among poor children, and evidence of the beneficial impact of increased access to medical care, it appears justifiable to conclude that medical care does reduce the frequency of occurrence of DKA; it does so by facilitating the management of acute nondiabetic illnesses that would otherwise precipitate acidosis in diabetic children.

References

Colle E, Siemiatycki J, West R, et al. Incidence of juvenile onset diabetes in Montreal: demonstration of ethnic differences and socio-economic class differences. J Chronic Dis 1981;34:611–16.

Connell F, Louden J. Diabetes mortality in persons under 45 years of age. Am J Public Health 1983;73:1174–77.

Davidson J, Delcher H, Englund A. Spin-off cost/benefits of expanded nutritional care. J Am Diet Assoc 1979;75:250–57.

Faich G, Fishbein H, Ellis S. The epidemiology of diabetic acidosis: a population based study. Am J Epidemiol 1983;117:551–58.

Fishbein H, Faich G. Epidemiology of insulin-dependent diabetes mellitus (DDM): the Rhode Island registry. Proceedings for the 5th Annual Diabetes Control Conference, Lexington, Kentucky, May 10–13, 1982:13–18.

Fishbein H, Faich G, Ellis S. Incidence and hospitalization patterns of insulin-dependent diabetes mellitus. Diabetes Care 1982;5:630–33.

Giordano B, Rosenbloom A, Heller D, Weber FT, Gonzalez R, Grgic A. Regional services for children and youth with diabetes. Pediatrics 1977;60:492–98.

Hoffman W, O'Neill P, Khoury C, Bernstein S. Service and education for the insulin dependent child. Diabetes Care 1978;1:285-88.

La Porte R, Orchard T, Kuller L, Wagener D, Drash A, Schneider B, Fishbein H. The Pittsburgh insulin dependent diabetes mellitus registry: the relationship of insulin dependent diabetes mellitus incidence to social class. Am J Epidemiol 1981;114:379-84.

Miller L, Goldstein J. More efficient care of diabetic patients in a county-hospital setting. N Engl J Med 1972;286:1388-91.

NDDG (National Diabetes Data Group). Selected statistics on health and medical care of diabetics 1980 (mimeo).

North AF, Gorwitz K, Sultz H. A secular increase in the incidence of juvenile diabetes mellitus. J Pediatr 1977;91:706-10.

Runyan J, VanderZwaag R, Joyner MB, Miller S. The Memphis diabetes continuing care program. Diabetes Care 1980;3:382-86.

Schade D, Eaton P. Prevention of diabetic ketoacidosis. JAMA 1979;242:2455-58.

Sultz H, Schlesinger E, Mosher W, Feldman J. Long-term childhood illness. Pittsburgh: Univ Pittsburgh Press, 1972:223-48.

13
Convulsive Disorders (Epilepsy): Prevention of Status Epilepticus

Barbara Starfield

Seizure disorders are uncommon but not rare in pediatric populations. Although the frequency of seizures themselves is not well documented, there is relative consistency in the estimates of the incidence and prevalence of seizure disorders. Figure 12 indicates that the incidence of seizure disorders is high in the first year of life, falls in childhood and adulthood, then rises again after age 50. Although these data derive from a study done in Rochester, Minnesota, the findings for early childhood are almost identical to those from a study done in Oakland, California (USDHEW 1978). Thus it is likely that they are generalizable, at least to predominantly white, middle-class populations in the United States. Patterns of the incidence of epilepsy from these studies are similar to those reported from a general practice in Great Britain (Fry 1966, 158) and from Norway, Iceland, and Carlisle, England (USDHEW 1978), except for a leveling or a slight increase in incidence in early adolescence in these four studies. Prevalence estimates (individuals with seizure disorders) vary widely but generally range between 4 and 12 per 1,000 children under age 21 (USDHEW 1978, Table 8). These data are consistent with prevalence data from a general practice in Great Britain: 8.5 per 1,000 children under age 10 (Fry 1966, 157).

Prevalence rates obtained from household interviews of individuals in the National Health Survey are somewhat lower (2.9 per 1,000 children under age 17). Although the number of children in this survey is too small to permit stable estimates of the relationship between prevalence and socioeconomic status, prevalence rates at ages 17–44 and 45 years and older decrease with increasing family income; they also decrease with increasing educational level of the head of the family in all age groups (NCHS 1977, 33). Moreover, increases in death rates are associated with social and environmental factors (Rodin 1972). Individuals with epilepsy had higher death rates in each age group up to age 45 than was the case for nonepileptics: 18.8 versus 14.8 at

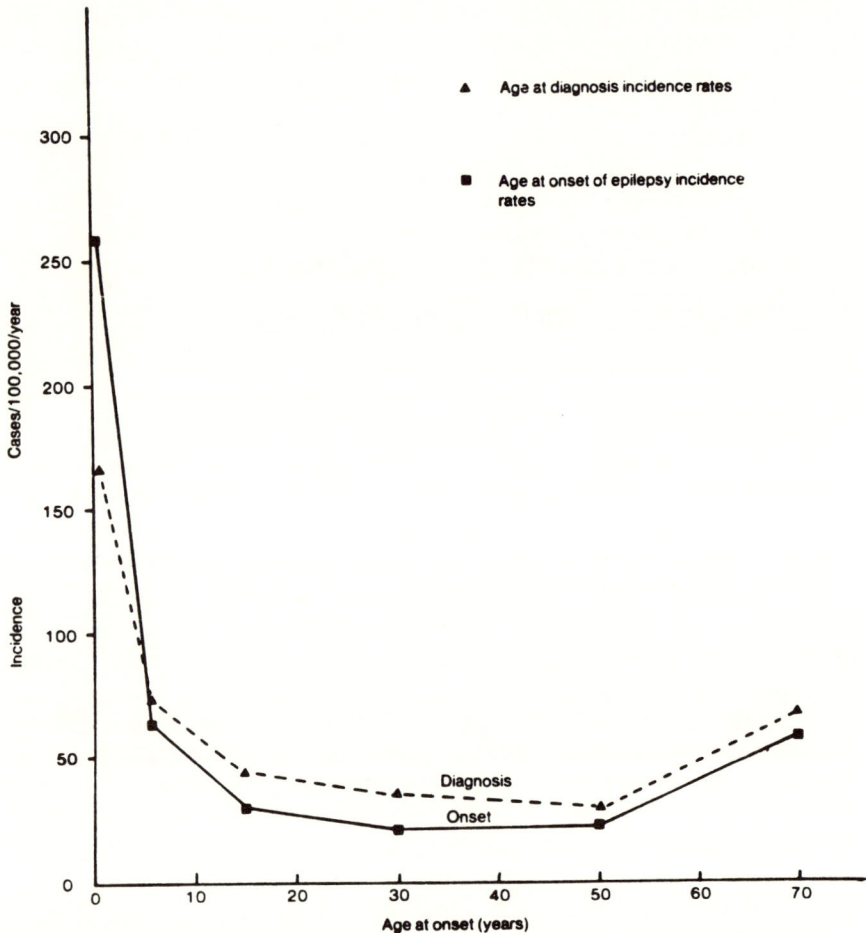

Figure 12. Incidence of Epilepsy in Rochester Study (Average Values for 1935–64 Period)*
Source: USDHEW 1978, 43.
*Data from Hauser and Kurland 1975

ages 0–5, 7.3 versus 1.1 at ages 5–24, and 11.4 versus 3.1 at ages 25–45 (Lennox 1960).

Studies of the incidence, prevalence, distribution, and prognosis of epilepsy are fraught with problems due to the lack of a standard definition of epilepsy, appropriate periods of follow-up, and variations in the types of seizures included in the framework of study. In general, an individual must have had at least two seizures in order to be labeled by investigators as a victim of seizure disorder, and most researchers eliminate seizures associated only with fever and those that result from injury or as a concomitant of other conditions. Given a representative group of people with one seizure, approximately one third will have no further seizures (USDHEW 1978). Although nomenclature varies from place to place and over time there are at least six widely diverse types of primary seizure disorders, each with its own type of therapy.

Status epilepticus is a state in which a seizure occurs for a prolonged period (more than 20 minutes for generalized tonic-clonic seizures) or when there is not total regain of consciousness between episodes lasting more than 30 minutes (Barbosa and Freeman 1982). In children, approximately half of the episodes of status epilepticus are associated with central nervous system pathology ("symptomatic"), particularly infections, metabolic disease, or chronic encephalopathy due to cerebral injury of developmental or idiopathic origin. Among the remainder, about half ("cryptogenic") are associated with fever and occur in children between 6 months and 3 years of age (Aicardi and Chevrie 1970). Although there is indication that reported rates of unfavorable sequelae that are derived from clinic-based studies are higher than those that would be obtained from studies in more representative populations (Ellenberg and Nelson 1980), these reports suggest that 3–8 percent of individuals with epilepsy will experience at least one episode of status epilepticus in their lifetime, with an estimated mortality of 6–18 percent. The occurrence of neurologic sequelae is reported to be even higher (Barbosa and Freeman 1982). In their study of all patients under 15 years of age hospitalized or seen as outpatients for status epilepticus at the Clinique de Pediatrie et Puericulture, Paris, from 1961 to 1968, Aicardi and Chevrie (1970) found that over three fourths (77 percent) of all instances of status epilepticus occurred in patients without a history of prior seizure. Symptomatic seizures due to acute causes were almost always the first seizure (and hence probably not preventable). Other types of symptomatic seizures were usually preceded by other episodes (and hence at least theoretically preventable if therapy were efficacious). Cryptogenic seizures were either the first convulsive attack or were preceded by one to three prior episodes. Unfortunately, Aicardi and Chevrie did not indicate whether febrile seizures (which are less amenable to prevention) were the type primarily seen in the first such episodes, or the extent to which the nonfebrile cryptogenic seizures were repeat or first episodes, so it is impossible to judge the potential preventability of cryptogenic seizures as a group.

There is, however, little doubt of the effectiveness of medical care for individuals with seizure disorders, even in the absence of controlled clinical trials (which now would be considered unethical). Longitudinal trends in prevalence of seizures would be difficult to interpret, even if data on prevalence of seizures were available, because of the variety of types of seizures and their differing response to a wide variety of therapies becoming available at different times. Therefore, evidence of the effectiveness of medical care is provided by three types of studies: those examining the pattern of recurrence of seizures after medication is withdrawn; those relating adequacy of therapeutic levels of medication with adequacy of control of seizures; and those addressing the relationship between access to care and seizure status.

Several studies have documented the safety of withdrawing medication in individuals who have been seizure-free after several years. Two of these have followed child patients sufficiently long to be considered definitive, and their findings are similar. Emerson et al. (1981) found that 70 percent of patients followed for an average of 27 years from whom medication had been withdrawn remained seizure-free. Of the 30 percent who did not, 78 percent of relapses occurred during the first year after withdrawing medication. Thurston et al. (1982) conducted a study that followed patients for at least 15 years after withdrawal of medications. Three quarters (76 percent) remained seizure-free. Of those who relapsed, 56 percent did so within one year. In both studies, all eligible patients in the facilities (which were service clinics in major medical centers) were included in the study and follow-up was complete (100 percent), even in Thurston's long-term study. Relapse was associated with conditions that were initially more severe (greater duration of seizures before control, severity of type of seizure, or number of seizures before control). Although the proportion of children with seizures that cannot be controlled is not reported and undoubtedly varies from place to place, in these two studies 32 percent and 6 percent of the children, respectively, became free of seizures by persistent attempts at medical control that took six years or longer to achieve.

Within the most recent decade, it has become possible to measure serum levels of anticonvulsants in the therapy of epilepsy. Two studies indicate that adequacy of blood levels is associated with better seizure control. Dawson and Jamieson (1971) studied the first 30 children who were receiving phenytoin and who were admitted to a hospital or appearing as an outpatient. These children, aged 6 months to 12 years, were followed for six months. Seven patients had therapeutic blood levels throughout the period; only one continued to have seizures. Ten of the other 23 patients were seizure-free at intake to the study, despite low blood levels. Of the 13 patients with inadequate levels and with convulsions, 11 were free from seizures after attaining therapeutic blood levels; the 2 patients with continuing convulsions failed to attain therapeutic levels. In a study of 70 individuals (mean age 12 years, range 4–28 years) with petit mal seizures (Sherwin et al. 1973), the clinical control of seizures significantly improved along with raised blood ethosuximide levels. At initiation of the study, patients with suboptimal blood levels of the drug were much more likely to be experiencing convulsions than patients with adequate levels. The percent of patients controlled rose from 64 to 81 percent with appropriate adjustment of blood drug levels. In 7 of 19 patients with improved blood levels, the increase was due to larger doses; in 10 it was due to better cooperation in taking medication; in 2 patients both factors were important. Thirteen of the 19 patients with improved drug levels improved clinically; 10 became seizure-free.

Although the above studies were done in facilities specializing in the management of epilepsy and therefore the findings may not be generalizable to the entire population, they do indicate that therapy is effective at least in the subgroup of patients followed in these facilities. Moreover, evidence for effectiveness of medical management is also found in the few community studies that have been done. Stifler (1957), in a study of the prevalence of epilepsy in Maryland prior to the 1960s, found that the four counties without local clinics for the diagnosis and management of epilepsy had much lower reported prevalence of epilepsy than counties with such clinics. Counties with clinics had identified 34 percent of the expected number of epileptics in the county; counties without such clinics had identified less than half this proportion (14.5 percent). As there was no reason to believe that the prevalence of epilepsy varied from county to county, Stifler concluded that the unavailability of the clinics led to an underdiagnosis (and hence inadequately controlled epilepsy) in the population of those counties.

A recent community-based study in Baltimore confirmed the benefits of certain aspects of medical care for epileptics. Sixty-seven students aged 12–20 with epilepsy were identified through their involvement with an epilepsy counseling program sponsored by the Baltimore City Schools; 126 controls were randomly selected from the same school system. Information was obtained through the use of a questionnaire that included a measure of psychological well-being validated for adolescents (The Offer Self Image Questionnaire). There were no differences in psychological well-being between adolescents with epilepsy and controls. Students with epilepsy had fewer psychosomatic complaints but were less likely to have a driver's license. Multiple regression analysis, however, showed that the best predictor of psychological well-being among students with epilepsy was knowledge about epilepsy. Frequency of seizures, age of onset, or perceived severity of epilepsy had no effect on psychological well-being after knowledge was considered. These findings suggested that health care providers can influence the well-being of children with epilepsy by communicating knowledge about the disorder to them (Hall 1984).

In summary, evidence from the few studies that have been conducted indicates that medical care for epilepsy is effective. Provision of services for children with epilepsy improves the rate of diagnosis of the condition; medications control seizures when they are properly administered and monitored, and provision of information by practitioners improves the well-being of children who have the condition.

References

Aicardi J, Chevrie J. Convulsive status epilepticus in infants and children. Epilepsia 1970;11:187–97.

Annegers J, Hanser WA, Elveback L. Remission of seizures and relapse in patients with epilepsy. Epilepsia 1979;20:729–37.

Barbarosa E, Freeman J. Status epilepticus. Pediatrics in Review 1982; 4:185-90.

Dawson K, Jamieson A. Value of blood phenytoin estimation in management of childhood epilepsy. Arch Dis Child 1971;46:386-88.

Ellenberg J, Nelson K. Sample selection and the natural history of disease: studies of febrile seizures. JAMA 1980;243:1337-40.

Emerson R, D'Souza B, Vining E, Holden K, Mellits ED, Freeman J. Stopping medication in children with epilepsy: predictors of outcome. N Engl J Med 1981;304:1125-29.

Fry J. Profiles of disease: a study in the natural history of common disease. Edinburgh: E & S Livingstone, 1966;157-60.

Hall D. Psychological well being in adolescents with epilepsy. General Pediatrics Academic Development Program. Johns Hopkins Univ School of Medicine, 1984.

Hauser WA, Kurland LT. The epidemiology of epilepsy in Rochester, Minnesota, 1935 through 1967. Epilepsia 1975;16:1-66.

Lennox, W. Epilepsy and related disorders. Boston: Little, Brown, 1960.

Maryland Development Disability Council. Epilepsy in Maryland: an assessment of services and gaps in service. Report to the Developmental Disabilities Council, July 1, 1975.

NCHS (National Center for Health Statistics). Prevalence of chronic conditions of the genitourinary, nervous, endocrine, metabolic, and blood and blood-forming systems and of other selected chronic conditions. United States—1973. Washington, D.C., U.S. Government Printing Office, (DHEW publication no. (HRA) 77-1536).

Rodin E. Medical and social prognosis in epilepsy. Epilepsia 1972;13:121-31.

Sherwin A, Robb JP, Lechter M. Improved control of epilepsy by monitoring plasma ethosuximide. Arch Neurol 1973;28:178-81.

Stifler J. A review of the Maryland epilepsy program. Am J Public Health 1957;47:587-93.

Thurston J, Thurston D, Hixon B, Keller A. Additional follow-up of 148 children 15 to 23 years after withdrawal of anticonvulsant therapy. N Engl J Med 1982;306:831-36.

USDHEW. The commission for the control of epilepsy and its consequences: plan for nationwide action on epilepsy. vol. IV. Washington, D.C., U.S. Government Printing Office, 1978 (DHEW publication no. (NIH) 78-279).

14
Bacterial Meningitis: Prevention of Sequelae

Barbara Starfield and Alain Joffe

Bacterial meningitis is one of the more severe acute illnesses of childhood. The vast majority of cases result from infection by one of three organisms: Hemophilus influenzae, Neisseria meningitidis, and Streptococcus pneumoniae; together they account for 84 percent of all bacterial meningitis in children and adults, and for over 95 percent of bacterial meningitis in children (CDC 1979). Nearly 80 percent of all reported bacterial meningitis occurs in children under age 21; 70 percent occurs in children under 5 (CDC 1979). The age-specific incidence of reported cases is given in Table 5. Hemophilus influenzae (H. influenzae) is the most common type of meningitis in children under 4 years of age. Case fatality rates depend upon the type of meningitis; they vary from 7.1 percent for H. influenzae to 13.5 percent for Neisseria meningitidis to 28.2 percent for Streptococcus pneumonia (also known as D. pneumoniae).

The above data are derived from reporting by 38 states representing 67.8 percent of the U.S. population. Meningitis is not a reportable disease (although meningococcal illness is). However, since 1977, 38 states have voluntarily participated in the surveillance of bacterial meningitis conducted by the Centers for Disease Control (CDC). These and data from other studies conducted by epidemiologists at the CDC provide much better information about the distribution and characteristics of disease in the population than the variety of studies based upon admissions to individual institutions. On the basis of studies in which reporting in defined communities was compared with casefinding by review of vital statistics and medical record review, the CDC concluded that the incidence figures as reported in Table 5 represent about 30 percent of the actual incidence of bacterial meningitis in the United States.

The organisms that cause most cases of bacterial meningitis in children are contagious. Before the era of antibiotics, meningococcal meningitis often occurred in epidemics with frequent spread to adults as well as children; nonepidemic meningococcal meningitis is primarily a disease of childhood

Table 5
Age-Specific Incidence of Reported Bacterial Meningitis, United States, 1978
(per 100,000 population)

Age	Neisseria Meningitidis	Hemophilus Influenzae	Streptococcus Pneumoniae
3 mos.–1 yr.*	13	49	5
1–2 yrs.	5	16	1
3–4 yrs.	2	3	0.3
5–9 yrs.	0.7	0.6	0.2
10–19 yrs.	0.6	0.1	0.1

Source: CDC 1979.
Note: The CDC estimates that these rates are about 30 percent of the national incidence of culture-proven bacterial meningitis.
* Estimated from table 2 in CDC 1979.

(D Fraser, personal communication). The risk of acquiring severe Hemophilus illness in household contacts of a patient with Hemophilus meningitis is approximately the same as the risk of acquiring secondary meningococcal disease (0.2 percent in the month after exposure). The risk is higher (0.5 percent) for contacts under 6 years of age (CDC 1979).

Several studies have demonstrated an inverse relationship between socioeconomic status (as determined by characteristics of census tract of residence) and frequency of occurrence of bacterial meningitis (Fraser et al. 1973a; Fraser et al. 1974; Floyd et al. 1974; Fraser et al. 1975), particularly with regard to Hemophilus meningitis; for meningococcal meningitis the findings were not consistent. Although rates were higher in nonwhites than in whites (Feldman et al. 1976), the difference was in part explained by differences in socioeconomic status except for pneumococcal disease; the clearly higher incidence of pneumococcal disease in blacks is partly due to the greater susceptibility of individuals with sickle hemoglobin (found primarily in blacks) to pneumococcal illness. Even when sickle cell disease is accounted for, however, incidence rates are still five times higher among blacks than among whites.

In a recent review of the evidence on the relationship between socioeconomic status and meningitis, Norden (1982) concluded that the "precise role of socioeconomic factors in the risk of an individual developing H. influenzae meningitis cannot yet adequately be assessed, but it would appear that children from large families, living in areas with low income levels, with low education levels for the parents, with higher population density, and with relatively poor access to medical care are at greater risk for H. influenzae meningitis" (p. 265).

Although no data on the community prevalence of sequelae of bacterial meningitis are available, several studies of individuals admitted to individual institutions indicate that sequelae are not uncommon. Of 50 children who recovered from H. influenzae meningitis at Vanderbilt Children's Hospital, only 50 percent were normal; 9 percent had only behavior problems and 28 percent had overall significant handicaps including hearing loss (20 percent), language delay or disorder (15 percent), mental retardation (11 percent), abnormal motor development (7 percent), and seizures (5 percent). In several studies, the overall incidence of seizures requiring medication for at least several years was 2-8 percent. (Some children had more than one of these complications [Sell 1983].) In ten studies with long-term follow-up and data on handicaps, the prevalence of sequelae from H. influenzae meningitis ranged from 8 percent (in those with follow-up of no longer than two years) to 37.5 percent (in those followed for longer periods of time) (Ferry et al. 1982). In a study of 86 children admitted in 1977-79 to Baylor affiliated hospitals in Houston with meningococcal meningitis, 27 percent experienced one or more significant complications, including vasculitis or arthritis occurring as allergic sequelae. Nearly one in five children (17 percent) had nonallergic sequelae including deafness, myocarditis, suppurative arthritis, or subdural effusions or empyema (Edwards and Baker 1981).

Of the 79 children (ages 0-17) admitted with pneumococcal meningitis to the Montreal Children's Hospital from 1948 to 1973, convulsions occurred in 26, coma in 7, cranial neuropathies in 3, and dehydration in 3. Over half of the 28 patients without predisposing conditions who were followed up had sequelae including deafness (11 percent), hydrocephalus (11 percent), convulsions (7 percent), mental retardation (7 percent), strabismus (4 percent), and behavior problems (4 percent). Unfortunately the extent to which more than one sequelae was present in individual patients was not stated, and the interval of time to follow-up was not mentioned. However all patients with deafness had complications noted during the acute course (Laxer and Marks 1977).

Except for prophylaxis that interrrupts the spread of meningitis there is little evidence that meningitis can be prevented. Although vaccines against pneumococcus and Hemophilus influenzae are being tested, there is as yet no evidence to indicate their effectiveness in reducing the incidence of meningitis. Focal infections (such as otitis) that are treatable are not common precursors of meningitis (Smith et al. 1982; Feigin and Dodge 1976). Although the Hemophilus influenzae organism is a common cause of otitis media, sinusitis, and conjunctivitis, the strains causing these conditions are nontypable or nonencapsulated and are present in 50-80 percent of well individuals. In contrast, the strains associated with meningitis (2-4 percent upper respiratory tract carrier rates) are type b encapsulated; occasionally these strains are associated with otitis or pneumonia (Turk 1982). In a review of the medical records of patients with symptomatic exudative H. influenzae-associated otitis media, Howie and Ploussard (reported in Harding et al. 1973, 25) found that 40 (22 percent) had 76 recurrent infections. In four children, recurrent infection was followed by meningitis or septicemia. (In all of these, otitis was associated with a type b strain; 14 percent of type b otitis media led to systemic infection.) Thus, although meningitis does follow from otitis media (and can therefore theoretically be prevented by adequate treatment of otitis), most cases of meningitis do not derive primarily from antecedent conditions.

Availability of medical care, however, may decrease the frequency of occurrence of meningitis by interrupting the spread of disease from primary cases to contacts. Attack rates in households and day care centers are much higher than in the general population. In household contacts of children with Hemophilus influenzae meningitis, attack rates are 3.8 percent among children under age 2, 1.5 percent among children ages 2–3, and 0.1 percent among children ages 4–5; these rates are approximately 600 times greater than those in the general population. Fifty percent of associated cases occur within three days of onset in the index case and 75 percent within seven days. Attack rates in day care centers are 1 percent in children under 4 years of age (CDC 1982). As the efficacy of prophylactic antibiotics (rifampin) has not been conclusively demonstrated, close surveillance of young contacts with prompt careful evaluation of febrile episodes is the primary mechanism to minimize the occurrence of secondary cases (Daum 1982).

Although trends in the case fatality rates in relationship to the emerging availability of efficacious therapy (antibiotics) might be thought to provide evidence of the effectiveness of medical care for meningitis, such analyses should be interpreted with great caution in the absence of incidence rates, because the denominator as well as the numerator of the rate may change with medical care availability.

In the study of 79 children with pneumococcal meningitis admitted to the Montreal Children's Hospital, the percentage who died fell from 19 percent during 1948 to 1962 to 3 percent from 1963 to 1973. The report of that study did not present data on the slope of the decline during or across the two time periods, so it is not possible to relate it to specific changes in medical care delivery that occurred from 1948 to 1973 (Laxer and Marks 1977).

Hemminki and Paakkulainen (1976) analyzed the rate of decline in mortality rates from several infectious diseases in Sweden and Finland, before the availability of antibiotics and afterward. The rate of decline was greater after the introduction of antibiotics for septicemia, meningitis other than meningococcal, and syphilis; no such change in trend was noted for meningococcal meningitis. Their analyses did not include documentation of incidence rates of the diseases.

Marked increases in the incidence of Hemophilus influenzae meningitis occurred in the United States between 1935 and the mid-1960s (Fraser 1982). In all studies but one (Michaels 1971), which was not population-based, incidence rates of H. influenzae meningitis have remained steady since the mid-1960s. Where there has been an increase in the frequency of occurrence of meningitis since that time, it has been associated with an increase in meningitis due to unusual organisms in older individuals (age 60 and older) (Floyd et al. 1974; Fraser et al. 1973b). Therefore, case fatality rates of meningitis might have declined prior to the mid-1960s as a result of an increase in the number of reported cases, which may have been due to increasing availability of medical care with increased rates of diagnosis and/ or the recognition of milder cases that have a lower likelihood of mortality. However, at least two studies, discussed below, have shown declines in case fatality rates in the absence of long-term changes in incidence rates.

In Olmsted County, Minnesota, the percentage of children of ages 1 month to 4 years with H. influenzae, D. pneumoniae, and N. meningitidis meningitis who died fell from 70 percent in 1935–46 to 14 percent in 1947–58 to 6 percent in 1959–70, whereas the incidence rates (cases per 100,000 population) in those years was 12, 9, and 40 for H. influenzae; 10, 5, and 7 for D. pneumoniae; and 2, 13, and 2 for N. meningitidis. The same was the case at other ages, but as ages 5–59 years were combined, it is not possible to determine the trends specifically for children above 5 years of age (Fraser et al. 1973b).

Finland and Barnes (1977) provide information on all patients with bacterial meningitis admitted to Boston City Hospital during selected years from 1935 to 1972. In their series, 21 percent of cases of D. pneumoniae, 71 percent of cases of N. meningitidis, and 93 percent of cases of H. influenzae were found in children ages 1–19, whereas only 45 percent of all cases of bacterial meningitis were in that age group. Table 6 presents findings calculated from data in their report, which included selected incidence ratios and years of introduction of specific antibiotics. Incidence ratios (cases per 1,000 admissions) of these three types of meningitis overall (and for all types) showed no trend over this time period. Survival rates, on the other hand, showed marked increases. The first increase (between 1935 and 1941) followed the introduction of sulfa drugs. Subsequent to the introduction of penicillin and streptomycin there was another increase (between 1941 and 1947). A third increase followed the introduction of chloramphenicol (1951 to 1953). Survival rates declined in the early 1960s (1961, 1963, and 1965) but increased thereafter (1969 and 1972) (Finland and Barnes 1977). Although not noted in the report of this study, the last increase in survival rates occurred in the absence of an identifiable "technology"; it did, however, follow improved access to medical care that occurred as a result of the legislation of 1965 and the implementation of programs such as Medicaid, Title V programs, and community health centers.

Several retrospective studies have indicated that delay in receipt of medical care is associated with an increased likelihood of sequelae and complications. Belsey et al. (1969) conducted a case-control analysis of 102 infants and children with bacterial meningitis admitted to the Tulane and Louisiana State University services of the Charity Hospital in New Orleans in 1963–64. All deaths and nearly all complications (neurologic, subdural effusions, altered state of consciousness greater than seven days) occurred in patients

Table 6
Incidence Ratio and Survival for Patients with Streptococcus Pneumoniae, Neisseria Meningitidis, and Hemophilus Influenzae Meningitis, Boston City Hospital, 1935–72

Year	Incidence Ratio (per 1,000 admissions)	Survival (%)	Year	Incidence Ratio (per 1,000 admissions)	Survival (%)
1935	.76	6.7	1957	.83	89.3
1941	.81	40.0	1961	1.01	62.5
1947	1.29	52.0	1963	.88	69.0
1951	.92	50.0	1965	.95	51.6
1953	.87	72.7	1969	.86	72.7
1955	1.0	68.6	1972	.66	71.4

Source: Finland and Barnes 1977.

who had either severe illness on admission or at least a three-day delay in hospitalization after the onset of symptoms compatible with meningitis. The proportion of patients with complications was 36.5 percent for survivors of H. influenzae meningitis, 60 percent for survivors of D. pneumoniae meningitis, and 9 percent for survivors of N. meningitidis meningitis. In another study reported from the same hospital, Belsey reported a significant relationship between delays of three days or more in the seeking of care and complications. In this study of 95 children ages 2 weeks to 6 years, delay in seeking care was present in 12 patients; 10 (83 percent) of these had high complication scores. In comparison, only 16 of 72 (22 percent) patients who did not delay in seeking care had high complication scores (Belsey 1969).

In a study of 86 children with meningococcal meningitis at Baylor-affiliated hospitals in 1977–1979, Edwards and Baker (1981) showed that the development of sequelae or complications was associated with severe illness on admission or fever greater than 38.3 degrees centigrade for longer than four days prior to admission.

Laxer and Marks (1977) stated that duration of symptoms before admission did not predict prognosis (mortality), but unfortunately no data were presented and their analysis did not control for other variables highly related to prognosis, i.e., age and year of diagnosis. They did indicate, however, that the accuracy of the diagnosis of the referring physician was probably related to prognosis; in their study the accuracy of diagnosis was much greater than in other studies that had higher mortality rates. Again, however, these analyses were not controlled for age or year of diagnosis. Feigin and Dodge (1976) reported that the presence of focal neurologic signs correlated significantly with delay in diagnosis in their study of 88 consecutive children (ages 2 months to 15 years) with bacterial meningitis. The presence of focal signs (in 13.6 percent of children) was correlated with the presence of sequelae detectable six months after hospital discharge. In this analysis, no attempt was made to control for other factors (such as age) that may have been associated with complications or sequelae.

In a Swiss study of 97 children ages 3 months to 8 years, Richner et al. (1979) showed that the interval between the appearance of initial symptoms and the start of therapy had a decisive and statistically significant influence on the incidence of hearing loss as measured several years later. When the delay was less than 48 hours, the incidence was 2 percent; when it was more than 48 hours, the incidence of subsequent hearing loss was 86 percent. In contrast to the authors of other studies, these authors demonstrated that age did not account for the difference, and the relationship between age and delayed care was independent both of the type of treatment received (ampicillin vs. chloramphenicol) and the presence or absence of otitis media.

Kresky et al. (1962) examined 80 children three to five years after discharge from Meadowbrook Hospital with diagnoses of bacterial meningitis in 1951–55. Over one third (34 percent) had neurologic deficits including convulsions, mental retardation, spasticity, poor coordination, facial weakness or sensory defect. Of children whose care was delayed for three or more days, 47 percent had subsequent deficit as compared with 10 percent for those receiving care within one day after onset of illness. Severity of illness in the hospital (as measured by length of stay) was associated with sequelae: 65 percent of those hospitalized over three weeks had sequelae as compared with 25 percent for those hospitalized less than two weeks. There was no relationship between type of meningitis and sequelae. Although infants were slightly more likely to have sequelae than older children, no mention was made of the relationship between delayed care and age.

Alon et al. (1979) studied 72 children three to eleven years after discharge from Rambam Medical Center (Israel) in 1960–68. Examinations were inconclusive in 7. Of the remaining 65, 52 percent (34) had sequelae. In 38 percent the sequelae were neurologic. Infants under 6 months were more likely to have sequelae. A diagnosis made during the first three days of illness was associated with a significantly better outcome; 43 percent of children diagnosed early had sequelae compared with 81 percent of those diagnosed after 72 hours. Moreover, children with seizures during hospitalization were significantly more likely (80 percent) to have sequelae than those without seizures (40 percent). No mention was made of the relationship between age, delay in diagnosis, and sequelae although infants under 6 months with a history of seizures were more likely to have abnormal EEGs on follow-up; this was not the case for older children. In this study, infections with Streptococcus pneumoniae were more likely to have sequelae.

Emmett et al. (1980) compared children with Hemophilus influenzae meningitis with their siblings at least two years after discharge from the Mater Children's Hospital or the Royal Children's Hospital in Brisbane, Australia. All subjects had meningitis after the neonatal period and all were treated with antibiotics. Children with meningitis performed significantly worse than their siblings on neurologic tests although none of the abnormalities were severe. Although no data are provided in the report, the authors stated that there was a consistently significant relationship between shorter illness (as measured by duration of symptoms before admission) and scores on psychological tests.

In a study from 1973 to 1975 of 73 Colorado children of ages 6 weeks to 3 years who had H. influenzae meningitis, duration of symptoms for more than three days prior to admission was associated with an increase in complications; the report did not distinguish between sequelae during hospitalization or those ascertained three months later, nor did it control for age in examining the relationship between delayed care and morbidity (Herson and Todd 1977).

Most of the studies cited above agree that neither type of meningitis nor prior receipt of antibiotics (before hospitalization) was related to sequelae. A majority reported that age under 1 year was associated with a poorer prognosis. Almost all studies found that delay in receipt of care was associated with a greater likelihood of complications although at least one investigator (Sell 1983) has interpreted studies in animal models as evidence that pathological processes presumably causing sequelae are already present by the time meningitis is clinically apparent. Hearing loss has been found in children hospitalized early in the course of their illness so that it is part of the acute disease, at least in some children. (Dodge et al. 1984; Vienny et al. 1984). Most of the clinical evidence on other neurologic sequelae, however, indicates that early receipt of appropriate medical care is beneficial for at least some patients, and early diagnosis and prompt rehabilitation is important where there is hearing loss in order to prevent permanent severe disability.

Higher case fatality rates in disadvantaged populations (Floyd et al. 1974) and greater incidence of bacterial meningitis among the poor and uneducated (Fraser et al. 1974) have been interpreted as evidence for the adverse effects of barriers to early health care.

The most striking demonstration of the impact of medical care on bacterial meningitis derives from a study in Vermont by Fraser et al. (1975). In this study of the occurrence of bacterial meningitis and deaths from bacterial meningitis in children from 1967 to 1970, two medical care variables were significantly associated with predicted rates of meningitis. In children of all ages, rates of bacterial meningitis were higher in towns with higher rates of hospitalization overall. For children age 5 and over, rates of diagnosed meningitis were also higher in towns that had a general practitioner or internist. The frequency of diagnosis of acute meningitis of unknown cause (not specified as bacterial) in children of all ages was also diagnosed more commonly in towns that had a general practitioner or internist. Most significantly, towns with fewer recognized meningitis cases than expected had significantly greater rates of death from obscure causes in children 1–59 months of age. After ruling out several competing explanations for these phenomena, the authors concluded that the observations were consistent with the thesis that inadequacies in medical care availability and utilization in some Vermont towns were associated with an underdiagnosis of meningitis and case fatality rates comparable to those prior to the antibiotic era (80 percent).

This evidence of increased deaths when medical care is less available and evidence that delay in receipt of care is associated with increased likelihood of sequelae indicate the importance of medical care on the course of bacterial meningitis in children. Although case fatality rates have declined markedly in the most recent two decades, the proportion of survivors with sequelae, especially deficits in learning and cognitive functioning, is increasing (Ferry et al. 1982; Edwards and Baker 1981). Since, as Emmett et al. (1980) suggest, these particular deficits are most closely linked to delay in diagnosis, problems with access to medical care are still pressing today.

References

Alon V, Naveh Y, Gardos M, Friedman A. Neurological sequelae of septic meningitis. Isr J Med Sci 1979;15:512–17.

Belsey M. CSF glutamic oxaloacetic transaminase in acute bacterial meningitis. Am J Dis Child 1969;117:288–93.

Belsey M, Hoffpauir C, Smith M. Dexamethasone in the treatment of acute bacterial meningitis: the effect of study design on the interpretation of results. Pediatrics 1969;44:503–13.

CDC (Centers for Disease Control). Bacterial meningitis and meningococcemia—United States 1978. MMWR June 22, 1979; 28(4):277–79.

CDC (Centers for Disease Control). Prevention of secondary cases of Haemophilus influenzae type b disease, MMWR Dec. 24, 1982; 31(50): 672–80.

Daum R. Role of rifampin in the management of household contacts of patients with invasive haemophilus influenzae infections. In:Sell, Wright, eds., op. cit., 1982:299–307.

Dodge P, Davis H, Feigin R, Holmes S, Kaplan S, Jubelirer D, Stechenberg B, Hirsh S. Prospective evaluation of hearing impairment as a sequela of acute bacterial meningitis. N Engl J Med 1984;311:869–74.

Edwards M, Baker C. Complications and sequelae of meningococcal infections in children. J Pediatr 1981;99:540–45.

Emmett M, Jeffrey H, Chandler D, Dugdale A. Sequelae of haemophilus influenzae meningitis. Aust Paediatr J 1980;16:90–93.

Feigin R, Dodge P. Bacterial meningitis: newer concepts of pathophysiology and neurologic sequelae. Pediatr Clin North Am 1976;23:541–55.

Feldman R, Koehler R, Fraser D. Race-specific differences in bacterial meningitis deaths in the United States, 1962–1968. Am J Public Health 1976;66:392–96.

Ferry P, Culbertson J, Cooper J, Sitton A, Sell S. Sequelae of haemophilus

influenzae meningitis: preliminary report of a long-term follow-up study. In:Sell, Wright, eds., op. cit., 1982:111–17.
Finland M, Barnes M. Acute bacterial meningitis at Boston City Hospital during 12 selected years, 1935–1972. J Infect Dis 1977;136:400–415.
Floyd R, Federspiel C, Schaffner W. Bacterial meningitis in urban and rural Tennessee. Am J Epidemiol 1974;99:395–407.
Fraser D. Haemophilus influenzae in the community and home. In Sell & Wright, 1982:11–22.
Fraser D, Darby C, Koehler R, Jacobs C, Feldman R. Risk factors in bacterial meningitis: Charleston County, South Carolina. J Infect Dis 1973a;127:271–77.
Fraser D, Geil C, Feldman R. Bacterial meningitis in Bernalillo County, New Mexico: a comparison with three other American populations. Am J Epidemiol 1974;100:29–34.
Fraser D, Henke C, Feldman R. Changing patterns of bacterial meningitis in Olmsted County, Minnesota, 1939–1970. J Infect Dis 1973b;128:300–307.
Fraser D, Mitchell J, Silverman L, Feldman R. Undiagnosed bacterial meningitis in Vermont children. Am J Epidemiol 1975;102:394–99.
Harding A, Anderson P, Howie V, Ploussard J, Smith D. Hemophilus influenzae isolated from children with otitis media. In:Sell S, Karzon D, eds. Hemophilus influenzae: proceedings of a conference on antigen-antibody systems, epidemiology, and immuno-prophylaxis. Nashville: Vanderbilt Univ Press, 1973:22–25.
Hemminki E, Paakkulainen A. The effect of antibiotics on mortality from infectious diseases in Sweden and Finland. Am J Public Health 1976; 66:1180–84.
Herson V, Todd J. Prediction of morbidity in hemophilus influenzae meningitis. Pediatrics 1977;59:35–39.
Kresky B, Buchbinder S, Greenberg I. The incidence of neurologic residua in children after recovery from bacterial meningitis. Arch Pediatr 1962;79:63–71.
Laxer R, Marks M. Pneumococcal meningitis in children. Am J Dis Child 1977;131:850–53.
Michaels R. Increase in influenzal meningitis. N Engl J Med 1971; 285:666–67.
Norden C. Hemophilus influenzae type b. In:Evans A, Feldman H, eds. Bacterial infections of humans; epidemiology and control. New York: Plenum, 1982:259–73.
Richner B, Hof E, Prader A. Hearing impairment following therapy of haemophilus influenzae meningitis. Helv Paediatr Acta 1979;34:443–47.
Sell S. Long-term sequelae of bacterial meningitis in children. Pediatr infect dis 1983;2(2):90–93.
Sell S, Wright P, eds. Haemophilus influenzae: epidemiology, immunology, and prevention of disease. New York: Elsevier Biomedical, 1982.

Smith A, Daum R, Scheifele D, et al. Pathogenesis of Haemophilus influenzae meningitis. In: Sell, Wright, eds., op. cit., 1982:89-109.

Turk D. Clinical importance of haemophilus influenzae—1981. In: Sell, Wright, op. cit., 1982:3-9.

Vienny H, Despland P, Lütschg J, Deonna T, Dutoit-Marco M, Gander C. Early diagnosis and evolution of deafness in childhood bacterial meningitis: a study using brainstem auditory evoked potentials. Pediatrics 1984; 73:579-86.

15
Acute Appendicitis

Nancy Hutton and Barbara Starfield

Acute appendicitis is the most common reason for abdominal surgery in children (Janik and Firor 1979; Lansden 1963). The estimated annual incidence and rates of appendicitis in children less than 15 years of age for selected years between 1968 and 1980 are given in Table 7. A trend toward a lower rate of appendicitis in the pediatric age group over the last decade is suggested by the data. Comparable data are not available for years prior to 1968, but one study of appendicitis in children of ages 16 or younger hospitalized between 1959 and 1968 in the Grady Memorial Hospital in Atlanta showed no change in the number of cases seen in that hospital per year during the study period (Stone et al. 1971).

Appendicitis occurs in all age groups, with most cases occurring in early adolescence (Lansden 1963; Bower et al. 1981; Scher and Coil 1980; Detmer et al. 1981). Data from the National Health Survey reveal that 30 percent of all appendicitis cases during 1971 and 1972 were in children under age 15 (NCHS, various years). Males outnumber females in the incidence of acute appendicitis (Janik and Firor 1979; Bower et al. 1981; Scher and Coil 1980; Detmer et al. 1981; Graham et al. 1980; Marchildon and Dudgeon 1977). There was a dramatic reduction in the mortality rate during the first half of this century due to the development of standards for the surgical management of this disease, improvement in the quality and safety of general anesthesia, and recognition of the need for preoperative stabilization of febrile, dehydrated, and infected patients (Cantrell and Stafford 1955; Peltokallio and Tykka 1981). Cantrell and Stafford (1955) reported a decrease in overall case fatality rate for acute appendicitis from 7 percent to 1 percent from 1930 to 1954; this change was attributed to improvement in the successful management of patients with appendiceal perforation. The rates of perforation in all age groups were 36.3 percent from 1931 to 1939, 23.2 percent from 1939 to 1947, and 26.1 percent from 1947 to 1954. Throughout the period of their study, the case fatality rate for unperforated acute appendicitis was only 0.14 percent. In contrast, the case

Table 7
Annual Incidence and Rates of Appendicitis in Children Less Than 15 Years, United States, 1968, 1971, 1972, 1978, 1979, and 1980

Year	Total Population of Children Less Than 15 yrs.	Number of Children with Appendicitis (First Listed Diagnosis)	Rate of Appendicitis per 10,000 Children	Percentage of Children Hospitalized with First Diagnosis of Appendicitis	Percentage of All Appendicitis Diagnoses That Were in Children
1968	59,473,000	116,000	19.5	2.9	
1971	57,368,000	94,000	16.4	2.5	29.6
1972	56,609,000	104,000	18.3	2.7	31.4
1978	50,823,000	80,000	15.8	2.4	26.3
1979	50,092,000	70,000	14.0	2.2	24.6
1980	51,169,000	76,000	14.8	2.1	28.5

Sources: NCHS 1982a, b.

fatality rate for those with perforation was initially 10 percent and decreased over the twenty-five year period to 2.7 percent.

More recent reports show a continued decline in childhood mortality due to appendicitis (Janik and Firor 1979; Graham et al. 1980; Marchildon and Dudgeon 1977). This trend is confirmed by national mortality figures (Tables 8 and 9). In 1950, 2.0 per 100,000 died as a result of acute appendicitis. In 1960 this rate fell to 1.0 per 100,000, in 1968 to 0.7 per 100,000, and by 1977 it was 0.3 per 100,000 population. This decline occurred in all child age groups except infants less than 1 year old.

Despite this improvement in mortality rates, the rates of perforation in children with appendicitis do not appear to have changed over the last forty-five years (Janik and Firor 1979; Lansden 1963; Stone et al. 1971; Scher and Coil 1980; Graham et al. 1980; Marchildon and Dudgeon 1977; Foster and Edwards 1957). Table 10 shows that infants are most likely to have perforated by the time of correct diagnosis. The higher rates of perforation in very young children are usually explained by the nonspecific nature of the presenting symptoms of appendicitis in this age group coupled with the difficulty in successfully examining these patients. They constitute the group with the longest duration of symptoms prior to correct diagnosis (Graham et al. 1980; Foster and Edwards 1957). They are more likely to have generalized peritonitis and, therefore, to be more seriously ill than older children due to a decreased ability to localize infection (Foster and Edwards 1957). Although acute appendicitis is rare in infants (well under 1 percent of cases according to studies by Lansden 1963 and Bower et al. 1981), its morbidity and mortality are of great concern. No improvement in the outcome of appendicitis in very young children has been made in the last two decades. Older children are less likely to present with appendiceal perforation than infants. When they do perforate, they more frequently localize the infection in the right lower quadrant of the abdomen. There is no relationship between race or sex and likelihood of perforation (Scher and Coil 1980).

Children with perforation encounter more complications and stay in the hospital longer than children with acute appendicitis without perforation (Lansden 1963; Stone et al. 1971; Bower et al. 1981; Detmer et al. 1981; Foster and Edwards 1957; Savrin and Clatworthy 1979). The average length of hospital stay has decreased since 1936, but there has been a consistent difference between those with and without perforation (Table 11).

Delay in admission to hospital has been consistently associated with increasing likelihood of perforation. Cantrell and Stafford (1955) reported on their experience with appendicitis at the Johns Hopkins Hospital from 1928 through 1954. In this study of patients of all ages, 13 percent of those with perforation were diagnosed within 24 hours and 38 percent within 48 hours of onset of symptoms. In contrast, 62 percent of patients with appendiceal perforation were symptomatic for more than 48 hours prior to diagnosis. Although no data were presented in their report, these investigators indi-

Table 8
Deaths in Children Due to Appendicitis, United States, 1950–78

Year	Total for All Ages	Age Groups (years)					Total			
		Under 1	1–2	2–3	3–4	4–5	0–5	5–9	10–14	15–19
1950	3,080	19	26	44	61	32	182	126	116	128
1958	1,845	24	14	9	11	10	68	63	61	37
1959	1,837	19	9	9	12	15	64	88	59	55
1960	1,871	13	7	16	16	11	63	68	75	50
1961	1,819	19	16	16	16	10	77	63	62	40
1962	1,800	21	7	14	11	11	64	62	82	60
1963	1,749	22	8	13	12	8	63	54	56	40
1964	1,783	14	8	9	7	8	46	55	76	46
1965	1,694	15	11	7	7	15	55	60	58	48
1966	1,627	19	8	9	8	11	55	61	52	43
1967	1,526	11	9	2	9	7	38	30	42	39
1968	1,485	13	4	8	5	10	40	41	43	40
1969	1,407	17	4	5	3	8	37	44	46	38
1970	1,397	16	6	3	6	6	37	30	45	27
1975	822	11	2	1	3	3	20	18	21	20
1977	747	7	5	1	1	4	18	14	16	5
1978	735	5	3	6	3	4	21	14	18	15

Source: NCHS for the years 1950, 1958–70, 1975, 1977, 1978.

Table 9
Death Rates (per 100,000) in Children Due to Appendicitis, United States, 1950–78

Year	Total for All Ages	Age Group (years)				
		Under 1	1–4	5–9	10–14	15–19
1950	2.0	1.1*	—	—	—	—
1960	1.0	0.3	0.3	0.4**		0.3***
1961	1.0	0.4	0.4	0.3**		0.3***
1962	1.0	0.5	0.3	0.3	0.5	0.4
1963	0.9	0.5	0.2	0.3	0.3	0.3
1964	0.9	0.3	0.2	0.3	0.4	0.3
1965	0.9	0.4	0.2	0.3	0.3	0.3
1966	0.8	0.5	0.2	0.3	0.3	0.2
1967	0.8	0.3	0.2	0.1	0.2	0.2
1968	0.7	0.4	0.1	0.2	0.2	0.2
1969	0.7	0.5	0.2	0.2	0.2	0.2
1970	0.7	0.5	0.2	0.2	0.2	0.1
1975	0.4	0.4	0.1	0.1	0.1	0.1
1977	0.3	0.2	0.1	0.1	0.1	0.0
1978	0.3	0.2	0.1	0.1	0.1	0.1

Sources: NCHS for the years 1950, 1958–70, 1975, 1977, 1978.
Note: Rates are calculated by number of deaths due to appendicitis in that age group divided by total population in that age group.
* Rate for 0–4 year olds.
** Rate for 5–14 year olds.
*** Rate for 15–24 year olds.

Table 10
Percentage with Appendiceal Perforation by Age

Author	Study Dates	Age Group (years)				
		0–2	3–5	6–10	11–12	12–20
Foster and Edwards 1957	1936–55	80	58	52	21	
Lansden 1963	1954–59	40	36	20		15***
Graham et al. 1980	1954–76	68	61			
Janik and Firor 1979	1957–76	55*				
Savrin and Clatworthy 1979	1970–75	93	71	40		30***
Scher and Coil 1980	1976–78		40**			21***

* Percentage for 0–5 year olds.

** Percentage for 0–10 year olds.

*** Percentage for 11–20 year olds.

Table 11
Average Length of Hospital Stay for Acute Appendicitis in Children with and without Perforation

Author	Study Dates	Length of Stay (days)	
		Without Perforation	With Perforation
Foster and Edwards 1957	1936–45	7	19
	1946–55	5	12
Lansden 1963	1954–59	5.3	9.5
Bower et al. 1981	1974–79	3.8	11
Detmer et al. 1981	1978*	5.4	10.2

* Reported as means for all patients (children and adults).

cated that "the striking common features among the fatal cases were prolonged duration of the disease and the presence of generalized peritonitis" (p. 752).

The experience with childhood (under age 13) appendicitis at Vanderbilt University Hospital from 1936 through 1955 was reported by Foster and Edwards (1957). The likelihood of perforation increased progressively with increased delay in operation after onset of symptoms: 7 percent when the delay was less than 24 hours, 25 percent when it was 24–47 hours, 59 percent at 48–71 hours, 68 percent at 72–96 hours, and 91 percent at over 96 hours. Moreover there was no evidence that perforation occurred earlier in infants than in older children. That is, the much higher frequency of perforated appendix in infants is not a result of greater likelihood of perforation but rather a result of delay in receiving appropriate care. The incidence of perforation in children residing outside of Nashville was over 49 percent as compared with 24 percent for residents of Nashville, a finding that further suggests the importance of ready access to medical care.

In a study of 880 consecutive patients with acute appendicitis from 1954 to 1959 at the Children's Hospital in Akron, Ohio, Lansden (1963) found that simple acute appendicitis without complications had symptoms for an average of 30.2 hours prior to admission. In contrast those with perforation or abscess had a mean duration of symptoms prior to hospitalization of 71.4 hours.

Graham et al. (1980) reported their experiences with 155 children under age 6 with appendicitis at the Texas Children's Hospital in Houston from 1954 to 1976. In this study, the mean duration of symptoms (presumably including those for children whose parents delayed seeking medical attention before operation) was 102 hours at ages under 4 and 58 hours at ages 4–6. Delay in receiving a correct diagnosis was directly related to the likelihood of perforation. The rate of perforation increased from 8 percent for children who had symptoms for less than 20 hours to 51 percent for those with symptoms 20–40 hours, 74 percent for those with symptoms 40–60 hours, 84 percent for those symptomatic for 60–80 hours and 87 percent for

Table 12
Percentage of Appendicitis Cases with Perforation, by Family Income, Huntington, West Virginia, 1976-78

Family Income	Total Cases	Number with Perforation	Percentage
less than $10,000	34	12	35
$10,000–$15,000	136	30	22
$15,000–$20,000	30	4	13
over $20,000	2	0	0
Total	202	46	23

Source: Scher and Coil 1980.

those with symptoms longer than 80 hours. In both age groups, the likelihood of perforation was related to duration of symptoms.

Of 335 patients with acute appendicitis at one of two hospitals in West Virginia in 1976-1978, 56 percent were under age 20 (Scher and Coil 1980). The incidence of perforation was significantly greater among patients living more than 20 miles from the hospital, even though transportation was uniformly available and there were no differences in reported access to a telephone. However, patients with perforation were ill for a significantly longer period before seeking medical care than patients without perforation: 2.5 days vs 1.5 days. In this study, perforation rates were highest in families of lowest income and decreased with increase in family income (Table 12).

Other studies have also reported an association between delay in seeking or receiving appropriate care and perforation. Of 677 children (16 years or younger) with appendicitis at Grady Memorial Hospital in Atlanta in 1959-1968, there were 398 patients with gangrenous or perforated appendices; of these, 211 were admitted on their first visit to a physician. Over three fourths (76 percent) of children with perforated appendices had symptoms more than 36 hours as compared with 56 percent of children with gangrenous appendices and 17 percent of those with acute appendicitis without gangrene or rupture (Stone et al. 1971). Pantell and Irwin's study (1979) of changes in the number of appendectomies performed before and during an anesthesiologists' boycott in San Francisco also included an examination of the relationship between delay in seeking care and perforation. The likelihood of perforation increased progressively with increasing delay in admission after onset of symptoms. Perforation frequencies were 7 percent for delays of 0-11 hours, 8 percent at 12-23 hours, 15 percent at 24-35 hours, 23 percent at 36-47 hours, and 26 percent at 48 or more hours. In this study, 1 of 203 patients (0.5 percent) was in the age group 0-5 and 43 (21 percent) were 6-15 years old. Of the primarily adult patients studied by Peltokallio and Tykka (1981), perforation frequencies increased progressively with increasing duration between onset of symptoms and operation in this study in the Helsinki University Central Hospital in Finland.

This evidence indicates that delay in the seeking of care, as may occur with decreased access to care or imposition of barriers to care, would be expected to result in more advanced illness at presentation (Foster and Edwards 1957), including greater likelihood of perforation, especially in older children. Delay in seeking care would also be reflected in an increase in the average length of hospital stay for all children with acute appendicitis due either to more children having perforation or to those with perforation being more ill at the time of diagnosis. Given the generally stable rates of perforation over time, any increase would be attributable to delay in receipt of adequate medical care rather than to changes in the pathogenesis or natural progression of this disease. Any increase in mortality from childhood appendicitis would be clear evidence of deterioration in the early diagnosis and/or adequate management of the problem.

References

Bower RJ, Bell MJ, Ternberg JL. Controversial aspects of appendicitis management in children. Arch Surg 1981;116:885–87.

Cantrell JR, Stafford ES. The diminishing mortality from appendicitis. Ann Surg 1955;141:749–58.

Detmer DE, Nevers LE, Sikes ED. Regional results of acute appendicitis care. JAMA 1981;246:1318–20.

Foster JH, Edwards WH. Acute appendicitis in infancy and childhood: a twenty-year study in a general hospital. Ann Surg 1957;146:70–77.

Graham JM, Pokorny WJ, Harberg FJ. Acute appendicitis in preschool age children. Am J Surg 1980;139:247–50.

Janik JS, Firor HV. Pediatric appendicitis: a 20-year study of 1640 children at Cook County (Illinois) Hospital. Arch Surg 1979;114:717–19.

Lansden FT. Acute appendicitis in children. Am J Surg 1963;106:938–42.

Marchildon MB, Dudgeon DL. Perforated appendicitis: current experience in a children's hospital. Ann Surg 1977;185:84–87.

NCHS (National Center for Health Statistics). Inpatient utilization of short-stay hospitals by diagnosis—United States. Vital Health Stat, series 13: nos. 12, 16, 20, 55, 69; 1982a (DHEW publication no. (HSM)73-1763, 3/73; DHEW publication no. (HRA)75-1767, 7/74; DHEW publication no. (HRA)76-1771, 11/75; DHHS publication no. (PHS)81-1716, 8/81; DHHS publication no. (PHS)83-1730, 12/82.

NCHS (National Center for Health Statistics). Utilization of short-stay hospitals: annual summary for the United States, 1980. Vital Health Stat, series 13, no. 64, 1982b (DHHS publication no. (PHS)82-1725, 3/82).

NCHS (National Center for Health Statistics). Vital statistics of the United States. vol. II—Mortality, 1950, 1958–1970, 1975, 1977, 1978 (various years).

Pantell RH, Irwin CE. Appendectomies during physicians' boycott. JAMA 1979;242:1627–30.

Peltokallio P, Tykka H. Evolution of the age distribution and mortality of acute appendicitis. Arch Surg 1981;116:153–56.

Savrin RA, Clatworthy HW. Appendiceal rupture: a continuing diagnostic problem. Pediatrics 1979;63:37–43.

Scher KS, Coil JA. Appendicitis: factors that influence the frequency of perforation. South Med J 1980; 73:1561–63.

Stone HH, Sanders SL, Martin JD. Perforated appendicitis in children. Surgery 1971;69:673–79.

16
Asthma

Lawrence S. Wissow and Barbara Starfield

Asthma is a major cause of morbidity among children and its treatment a major drain on medical resources. Although mortality from asthma is low (0.5-3 per 100,000 per year) (Stolley 1972; Gordis 1973), asthma is responsible for about one third of all chronic illness in children and is a leading cause of missed school days caused by chronic conditions (Schiffer and Hunt 1963; Hindi-Alexander and Cropp 1981). Over half of school-aged children who wheeze are reported to miss some school time because of their condition (Anderson et al. 1983). Asthmatic children are frequent users of outpatient facilities. When they present with acute attacks of wheezing, as many as one in ten will be admitted to the hospital (Drachman 1983). In one series, asthmatic children accounted for 8 percent of all pediatric medical admissions to a large university hospital, and admission rates appear to be increasing (Palm et al. 1970; Anderson 1978). In the United States, the number of discharges per 10,000 population with a first listed diagnosis of asthma rose from 5.5 in 1971 to 10.9 in 1975, to 24.3 in 1980, and to 29.3 in 1982 (NCHS 1974, 1978, 1982). Estimates from the National Ambulatory Medical Care Survey (NCHS 1977) indicate that asthma accounted for about 729,000 visits to pediatricians alone, or 1.6 percent of all visits to pediatricians.

Epidemiologic study of asthma is complicated by a basic lack of knowledge about the etiology and pathophysiology of the disease. In addition, differences in case finding and definition make comparisons among studies difficult. One-year period prevalence for children in the U.S. is estimated to be about 3 percent, with slightly higher rates in the South, among nonwhites, and in low-income families (NCHS 1973). Prevalence rates, as reported in the Health Interview Survey in 1970 were 29.3 per 1,000 at ages under 6 and 32.0 per 1,000 at ages 6-16. Rates in children in the lowest income category were 32.9 and 38.4 in the two age groups, respectively. One-year prevalence rates of 7 to 10 percent have been found in school-age children when parents are asked about symptoms likely to be attributable to asthma (Mak et al. 1982; Lee et al. 1983).

Exposure to airborne irritants and certain foods and drugs has been thought to play a role at least in the induction of individual attacks of wheezing, but no decrease in prevalence has been noted in Great Britain as air quality has improved (NHLBI 1980). Some studies have found increases in school absence and general respiratory symptoms in children exposed to very high levels of air pollution, but the studies have methodological flaws and the pollution levels were generally above present-day standards (Holland et al. 1979). Differential effects of various air pollution components have not been well characterized (Perry et al. 1983). Although some attacks appear to be triggered by viral upper respiratory infections, these viral infections are not preventable at the current time (Lwoff 1983).

There is strong evidence that medical care can influence the prevalence of asthmatic symptoms. Several drugs, among them the theophylline derivatives, have been shown in controlled clinical trials to reduce frequency and severity of wheezing in asthmatic children (Weinberger and Bronsky 1974). Special education programs, home visits, and adherence to individually tailored drug regimens have been shown for small groups and for limited periods of time to reduce days of disability, numbers of acute attacks, and return visits to emergency services (Maiman et al. 1979; Fireman et al. 1981; Ekwo and Weinberger 1978). Inhalation of an adrenergic agent such as epinephrine or isoproterenol may be sufficient in controlling occasional attacks of mild wheezing and, for most patients adding optimal doses of an oral theophylline preparation (including sustained-release preparations) will achieve control with minimal adverse effects (Medical Letter 1982). Other drugs (such as Cromolyn) are useful for mild paroxysmal asthma in children, but patients with severe persistent symptoms may require systemic or inhaled corticosteroids (Medical Letter 1982). Variability in absorption and metabolism may require monitoring of serum concentrations of drugs by medical personnel (Medical Letter 1984). Although yearly measurements of serum concentrations are sufficient for adults after establishment of an optimal regimen, children require more frequent monitoring because of their growth and developmental changes and greater propensity to febrile illness that alters drug metabolism (Hendeles and Weinberger 1983). The need for care in achieving optimal levels of therapeutic drugs and for monitoring them suggests that access to appropriate medical care might be an important determinant of effective medical care for asthma.

In Great Britain, 34 percent of asthmatic children who had seen their family doctor in the past year had an effective antiasthmatic drug in their home, whereas only 14 percent of asthmatic children reporting no doctor contact had such medication. This difference persisted even after adjustment for severity of asthma (Anderson et al. 1981). In another English study, 39 percent of children who sought care directly from the emergency room for acute attacks of asthma were readmitted to the hospital in the same calendar year. In contrast, only 11 percent of children referred to the emergency room by their doctor required readmission after the initial referral. At the time of initial referral both groups had a similar duration of acute symptoms and the self-referred patients were considered to have less severe disease as manifested by a lower mean pulse rate (Anderson et al. 1980). In Baltimore, children who used the emergency room as their primary source of asthma care were reported to have higher hospitalization rates (23 vs. 11 percent hospitalized within the previous 12 months) than those who obtained care from a private pediatrician or clinic (Mak et al. 1982). In an urban, low-income population less than half the children reported by their parents to have asthma were said to receive regular care for the condition (medical attention at times other than acute attacks). Moreover, 45 percent of asthmatic children whose regular source of care was a health maintenance organization were reported to receive ongoing (nonacute) attention for their condition, as compared with 26 percent for a sample of children whose predominant source of routine care was a hospital outpatient clinic (German et al. 1976).

In both the United Kingdom and Australia, school surveys have found that a large proportion of wheezy children do not receive medical attention and that many are misdiagnosed as having nonspecific respiratory ailments. Lee and coworkers (1983) surveyed 2,700 7 year olds and identified 150 (9 percent) as having symptoms consistent with asthma at some time since starting school. Their survey instrument had been demonstrated to have a high sensitivity for known asthmatic children. Specificity was estimated by response (unblinded and uncontrolled) to subsequent administration of bronchodilators. Eighty-eight of 89 treated children reported improvement of symptoms and decreased frequency of attacks. Parents of only 19 of the 150 wheezing children reported they knew that their child had had asthma.

Failure of diagnosis was found to be associated with inadequate and inappropriate treatment. One third of children who reported more than 12 episodes of wheezing in the past three years had never had a bronchodilator prescribed. Children with undiagnosed wheezing were much more likely to have received antibiotics for episodes of respiratory distress than were those known to be asthmatic (85 vs. 5 percent). One quarter of those families having bronchodilator drugs on hand reported inadequate knowledge of their proper use, and many reported inadequate home management of potentially life-threatening episodes of respiratory distress. School absenteeism fell tenfold (over a follow-up period that was not clearly specified) in the 31 children with more than 12 episodes of wheezing, after continuous treatment was instituted (Speight et al. 1983).

In an Australian study, follow-up of asthmatic children at age 21 revealed that undertreatment and lack of knowledge of asthma, originally noted in childhood, had continued. Twenty percent who reported wheezing more than once a week had no regular source of care, nor did 49 percent of those with less frequent wheezing. The prevalence of smoking, felt to aggravate asthma and have synergistic negative effects on lung function, was actually higher in the frequent wheezers (52 percent) than controls (40 percent) (Martin et al. 1982).

The pattern of asthma deaths among persons of all ages suggests that a portion might be prevented by timely care or appropriate home medication. In one city in Great Britain, 102 of 143 asthma deaths occurred outside the hospital or upon arrival. Only 17 of the 143 had been wheezing for less than 30 minutes before death, and some of those who died at home had been wheezing for as long as two weeks. None of the patients who died after hospital admission had been wheezing for less than two hours. All but a small number of patients should have had time to use potentially life-saving medication at home or in a medical facility (MacDonald et al. 1976a, b). In a similar but more recent study in adults only, inadequate medical care and patient education were judged to be major contributing factors to mortality among the 86 percent of adult asthma deaths in a one-year period that were considered to be preventable (British Thoracic Association 1982). Ninety-nine adult asthma deaths occurring over a one-year period were reviewed by a panel of physicians. Fifty-five of the 90 were judged to have been prescribed medication in inadequate doses. Failure to appreciate the suddenness with which death in asthma can occur and to have appropriate home emergency medication available was judged to be the most important factor contributing to death. Physicians as well as patients and family members were responsible for these failures.

These studies suggest that among asthmatics who died, potentially efficacious treatment was never given a chance to work. That is, efficacious care was not provided to or used by a substantial proportion of individuals who died.

In summary, medical care is capable of modifying morbidity and mortality from asthma. The results of several studies confirm the importance of access to adequate ongoing care for the prevention of symptoms and disability from this condition.

References

Anderson HR. Increase in hospitalization for childhood asthma. Arch Dis Child 1978;53:295–300.

Anderson HR, Bailey PA, Cooper JS, Palmer JC. Influence of morbidity, illness label, and social, family and health service factors on drug treatment of childhood asthma. Lancet 1981;2:1030–32.

Anderson HR, Bailey PA, Cooper JS, Palmer JC, West S. Morbidity and school absence caused by asthma and wheezy illness. Arch Dis Child 1983;58:777–84.

Anderson HR, Bailey P, West S. Trends in the hospital care of acute childhood asthma 1970-78: a regional study. Br Med J 1980;281:1191-94.

British Thoracic Association. Deaths from asthma in two regions of England. Br Med J 1982;285:1251-55.

Drachman RC. Unpublished data from the CARE system, 1983.

Ekwo E, Weinberger M. Evaluation of a program for the pharmacologic management of children with asthma. J Allerg Clin Immunol 1978;61:240-47.

Fireman P, Friday GA, Gira C, Vierthaler WA, Michaels MS. Teaching self-management skills to asthmatic children and their parents in an ambulatory care setting. Pediatrics 1981;68:341-48.

German PS, Skinner EA, Shapiro S, Salkever DS. Preventive and episodic health care of inner-city children. J Community Health 1976;2:92-106.

Gordis L. Epidemiology of chronic lung diseases in children. Baltimore: Johns Hopkins Univ Press, 1973.

Hendeles L, Weinberger M. Improved efficacy and safety of theophylline in the control of airways hyperactivity. Pharmacol Ther 1983;18:91-105.

Hindi-Alexander M, Cropp GJ. Community and family projects for children with asthma. Ann Allergy 1981;46:143-148.

Holland WW, Bennett AE, Cameron IR, et al. Health effects of particulate pollution: reappraising the evidence. 5. exposure to particulate pollution: studies in children. Am J Epidemiol 1979;110:604-15.

Lee DA, Winslow NR, Speight AN, Wey EN. Prevalence and spectrum of asthma in childhood. Br Med J 1983;286:1256-58.

Lwoff A. Traiter le rhume par la chaleur. Le Monde, no. 1793, 1983.

MacDonald JB, MacDonald ET, Seaton A, William DA. Asthma deaths in Cardiff 1963-74: 53 deaths in hospital. Br Med J 1976a;2:721-23.

MacDonald JB, Seaton A, Williams DA. Asthma deaths in Cardiff 1963-74: 90 deaths outside hospital. Br Med J 1976b;1:1493-95.

Maiman LA, Green LW, Gibson G, MacKenzie E. Education for self treatment by adult asthmatics. JAMA 1979;241:1919-22.

Mak H, Johnston P, Abbey H, Talamo RC. Prevalence of asthma and health service utilization of asthmatic children in an inner city. J Allergy Clin Immunol 1982;70:367-72.

Martin AJ, Landau LI, Phelan PB. Asthma from childhood at age 21: the patient and his disease. Br Med J 1982;284:380-82.

Medical Letter. Drugs for asthma. New York: The Medical Letter, vol. 24, issue 618, Sept. 17, 1982.

Medical Letter. Sustained-release theophyllines. New York: The Medical Letter, vol. 26, issue 652, Jan. 6, 1984.

NCHS (National Center for Health Statistics). Prevalence of selected chronic respiratory conditions, United States—1970. Vital Health Stat, series 10, no. 84, 1973 (DHEW publication no. (HRA)74-1511).

NCHS (National Center for Health Statistics). Inpatient utilization of short-stay hospitals by diagnosis, United States 1971. Vital Health Stat, series 13, no. 16, 1974 (DHEW publication no. (HRA)75-1767).

NCHS (National Center for Health Statistics). Ambulatory medical care rendered in pediatricians' offices during 1975. Advance data no. 13, Oct. 13, 1977.

NCHS (National Center for Health Statistics). Inpatient utilization of short-stay hospitals by diagnosis, United States 1975. Vital Health Stat, series 13, no. 35, 1978 (DHEW publication no. (PHS)78-1786).

NCHS (National Center for Health Statistics). Utilization of short-stay hospitals: annual summary for the United States, 1980. Vital Health Stat, series 13, no. 64, 1982 (DHHS publication no. (PHS)82-1725).

NCHS (National Center for Health Statistics). 1982 summary: national hospital discharge summary. Advance data no. 95, Dec. 27, 1983.

NHLBI (National Heart, Lung, and Blood Institute). Task force report on epidemiology of respiratory diseases. Oct. 1980 (NIH publication no. 81-2019).

Palm CR, Murcek MA, Roberts TR, Mansmann HC, Fireman P. A review of asthma admissions and deaths at children's hospital of Pittsburgh from 1935 to 1968. J Allergy 1970;46:257–69.

Perry GB, Chai H, Dickey DW, et al. Effects of particulate air pollution on asthmatics. Am J Public Health 1983;73:50–56.

Schiffer C, Hunt E. Illness among children: data from U.S. National Health Survey, 1963. Children's Bureau (DHEW publication no. 405).

Speight AN, Lee DA, Hey EN. Underdiagnosis and undertreatment of asthma in childhood. Br Med J 1983;286:1253–56.

Stolley PD. Asthma mortality. Am Rev Respir Dis 1972;105:880–90.

Weinberger MM, Bronsky EA. Evaluation of oral broncho-dilator therapy in asthmatic children. J Pediatr 1974;84:421–27.

17
Gastroenteritis and Dehydration

Lawrence S. Wissow and Barbara Starfield

Acute gastroenteritis (diarrhea) is among the most important child health problems in the world. In developing countries, it interacts with malnutrition to cause about 5 million deaths a year and is the leading cause of childhood deaths in the world. Children may suffer one to two serious episodes a year with case-fatality rates of up to 4 percent (Rohde and Northrop 1976). Death rates from diarrheal disease in young children have declined sharply in Latin America in the last decade, but in some areas they remain 60 times higher than the death rate in North America. As recently as 1978, death rates in Latin American children less than 1 year of age ranged from 480 to 1,800 per 100,000 and in children less than 5 years old from 24 to 640 per 100,000 (CDC 1983).

While diarrheal illness in developing countries has received considerable attention and is the focus of major public health efforts (Sack 1982; Population Reports 1980), in developed countries the need for intervention has been questioned (Jackson 1983). Controversy results from the fact that most gastroenteritis is self-limited and well-tolerated in persons of good nutritional status and good general health (Gordon et al. 1963). Morbidity and mortality attributable to diarrheal illness in developed countries, however, remains substantial. There were over 700 deaths attributed to diarrheal disease in infants in the United States in 1978 (USDHHS 1982). Gastroenteritis continues to rank in the top ten causes of death for ages 1 to 4 in Europe and North America (Rohde and Northrop 1976; Richmond 1977). It also causes extensive morbidity in the developed world. In the United States, 15 percent of a cohort of infants had one or more episodes of diarrhea by the age of 17 months (O'Connor et al. 1980). In Great Britain, 2 to 3 percent of children in one birth cohort were hospitalized for gastroenteritis in the first five years of life (Taylor et al. 1982). In another study, the proportion of children hospitalized for diarrhea before their first birthday was 4 percent among an inner city cohort of minority-group children (Walker-Smith et al.

1983). Gastroenteritis may also predispose to subsequent morbidity. For example, in a cohort of healthy infants followed until age 10 months, 13 of 62 episodes of diarrhea were followed by a fall-off in normal weight gain; it took up to two months for recovery of normal weight gain (Cushing and Anderson 1982). Some groups of children are at particularly high risk of diarrheal illness. It is estimated that at least 5 million children between the ages of 3 and 5 years attend day care centers. These facilities have become the site of diarrhea epidemics where attack rates of up to 80 percent have been reported (Pickering and Woodward 1982). Attack rates for infant "summer diarrhea" on Indian reservations have been reported to be as high as 40 percent during a study period of only 13 weeks, with up to 20 percent of ill children requiring hospital care (Woodward et al. 1974). Migrant worker populations are also at risk because of poor sanitary conditions and lack of medical care. In an epidemic of diarrhea in a Maryland migrant camp, the age-specific attack rate for children less than 1 year old was 89.2 percent. The mean age of 90 individuals who were taken ill was 15 months; eleven were hospitalized and one infant died (Maryland 1982).

Public health measures such as sanitation and refrigeration have been the mainstay of primary prevention, that is, prevention of the occurrence of gastroenteritis. Vaccines for rotaviral and some forms of bacterial diarrheas are under development but are not yet available (Levine and Edelman 1979). The introduction of fluid therapy has been credited with the dramatic improvement in secondary prevention, that is, the reduction in morbidity and mortality from gastroenteritis (Gordon et al. 1963; Gordon 1971).

Medical evaluation and specific supportive care are recommended for all but the most transient of diarrheal episodes (DeAngelis 1979; Shirkey 1980; Nelson 1979) in order to reduce costs, disability, and need for hospitalization (Medical Letter 1983; Finberg et al. 1982). The early treatment of gastroenteritis can be expected to reduce disability and discomfort and prevent hospitalization and other serious sequelae (Sack 1982) while maintaining caloric intake to avoid weight loss (Rohde and Northrop 1976; Brown and MacLean 1984). These goals are approached by the early provision of replacement and maintenance fluids, the identification of treatable causes and concurrent illness, and prompt resumption of appropriate feedings. Such therapy requires both physical and laboratory examination of the sick child as well as education for the child's caretaker. Caretakers must learn to assess fluid losses in stools, signs of dehydration, and cues for refeeding. They must also learn appropriate ways of providing nutrition and hydration. Homemade rehydration solutions, unless prepared with specific instructions, are likely to be inappropriate in salt and glucose content (Sack 1982), and simple "clear liquids" recommended by many sources on child care are not appropriate when diarrhea persists for more than 48 hours (Katz and Hyams 1980).

Advances in diagnostic techniques have made medical examination more important from both individual and public health perspectives. Pathogens can be determined in from 50 to 80 percent of cases, depending on the laboratory resources available (Edelman and Levine 1980). Different pathogens may require different treatment: rotaviral infection may require a different refeeding plan (Brown and MacLean 1984); pathogenic bacteria and protozoa may cause conditions that are not self-limited and require specific therapy (Wittner 1980). Especially when infected children spend time in day care centers or schools, identification of a particular pathogen may be important to the prevention of epidemics. Many such institutions have inadequate facilities for reducing the spread of diarrheal illness (Pickering and Woodward 1982).

As recently as 1946, the death rate for infants hospitalized with diarrhea was over 30 percent as demonstrated by a study done at the Johns Hopkins Hospital (Govan and Darrow 1946); within a few years it fell to less than 5 percent (Hirschhorn 1980) largely because of improvements in the management of infants hospitalized with acute gastroenteritis. Intravenous (Nalin 1972) and subsequently oral fluid therapies have been shown to markedly reduce case fatality rates in areas of endemic diarrhea (Oral glucose 1975; Rahman et al. 1979; Mahalanabis et al. 1973). In developed countries, studies in hospitalized patients have demonstrated the efficacy and safety of oral treatment and its advantages over intravenous therapy (Santosham et al. 1982). In outpatient trials in the Philippines, children in villages receiving oral therapy had better annual weight gain and smaller weight loss per episode of diarrhea than children in other villages (WHO 1977). Oral therapy can adequately replace intravenous solutions for most patients not yet in shock, and it can do this with minimal medical supervision in a wide variety of diarrheal illnesses and in children of developed as well as undeveloped countries (Santosham et al. 1982; Pizarro et al. 1983).

Along with monitoring of growth, expanded immunizations, and support for breast feeding, oral rehydration has become a major part of the UNICEF world-wide program to promote child health. Child mortality rates have been halved in several countries where the rehydration component of the program was implemented. Death rates also fell in hospitalized patients when oral therapy was substituted for intravenous therapy. In Costa Rica, the cost savings attributed to this switch was estimated to be about $3 million (Grant 1984).

Evidence for effectiveness of medical care for acute gastroenteritis is largely inferred from the abundant evidence of efficacy or from studies of effectiveness in developing countries as noted above. However, there is at least one study that demonstrates the importance of appropriate access to services in developed countries. McDonald et al. (1974) showed that the seeking of care for diarrhea is income dependent. The effect of income could be overcome, however, by facilitating access to medical care. Before the institution of universal health insurance in a Canadian province, care was sought for only 56 percent of low-income children with diarrhea of more than one day's duration, compared to 66 percent of children in families with higher incomes. After institution of universal health insurance, the percentage of children for whom care was sought rose to 74 in both groups.

In summary, access to appropriate medical care can be expected to reduce morbidity and mortality associated with diarrheal disease.

References

Brown KH, MacLean WC, Jr. Nutritional management of acute diarrhea: an appraisal of the alternatives. Pediatrics 1984;73:119-25.

CDC (Centers for Disease Control). Diarrheal diseases control program in the Americas. MMWR 1983;32:73-75.

Cushing A, Anderson L. Diarrhea in breast-fed and non breast-fed infants. Pediatrics 1982;70:921-25.

DeAngelis C. Pediatric primary care, 2d ed. Boston: Little Brown, 1979: 281-83.

Edelman R, Levine MM. Acute diarrheal infections in infants. II: bacterial and viral causes. Hosp Pract 1980;Jan.:97-104.

Finberg L, Harper PA, Harrison HE, Sack RB. Oral rehydration for diarrhea. J Pediatr 1982;101:497-99.

Gordon JE. Diarrheal disease of early childhood—worldwide scope of the problem. Ann NY Acad Sci 1971;176:9-15.

Gordon JE, Chitkara ID, Wyon JB. Weanling diarrhea. Am J Med Sci 1963;245:345-77.

Govan CD, Jr, Darrow DC. The use of potassium chloride in the treatment of the dehydration of diarrhea in infants. J Pediatr 1946;28:541-49.

Grant JP. The state of the world's children, 1984. Oxford: Oxford Univ Press, 1984.

Hirschhorn N. The treatment of acute diarrhea in children: an historical and physiological perspective. Am J Clin Nutr 1980;33:637-63.

Jackson W. Oral rehydration, diarrhea, and general practice. (letter) Lancet 1983;1:178.

Katz AJ, Hyams J. Gastrointestinal disorders. In: Graef JW, Cone TE, eds. Manual of pediatric therapeutics, 2d ed. Boston: Little Brown, 1980.

Levine MM, Edelman R. Acute diarrheal infections in infants. I: epidemiology, treatment, and prospects for immunoprophylaxis. Hosp Pract 1979;Dec.: 89-100.

McDonald AD, McDonald JC, Salter V, Enterline PE. Effects of Quebec medicare on physician consultation for selected symptoms. N Engl J Med 1974;291:649-52.

Mahalanabis D, Choudhuri AB, Bagchi NG, Bhattacharya AK, Simpson

TW. Oral fluid therapy of cholera among Bangladesh refugees. Johns Hopkins Med J 1973;132:197-205.

Maryland, State of, Department of Health and Mental Hygiene. Diarrheal outbreak in a migrant camp. Division of Communicable Diseases and Epidemiology Newsletter, Sept. 1982.

Medical Letter. Oral rehydration solutions. Medical Letter 1983;25:19-20.

Nalin DR. Mortality from cholera and other diarrheal diseases at a cholera hospital. Trop Geogr Med 1972;24:101-10.

Nelson WE, Vaughan VC, McKay RJ, Behrman RE. Nelson's Textbook of Pediatrics, 11th ed. Philadelphia: Saunders, 1979:1072-74.

O'Connor S, Vietze PM, Sherrod KB, Sandler HM, Altemeir WA. Reduced incidence of parenting inadequacy following rooming in. Pediatrics 1980;66:176-82.

Oral glucose/electrolyte therapy for acute diarrhea. Lancet 1975;1:79-80.

Pickering LK, Woodward WE. Diarrhea in day care centers. Pediatr Infect Dis 1982;1:47-52.

Pizarro D, Posada G, Mata L. Treatment of 242 neonates with dehydrating diarrhea with an oral glucose-electrolyte solution. J Pediatr 1983; 102:153-56.

Population Reports. Oral rehydration therapy for childhood diarrhea. Popul Rep [L], no. 2, Nov.-Dec., 1980.

Rahman MM, Aziz KMS, Patwari Y, Munshi MH. Diarrheal mortality in two Bangladeshi villages with and without community-based oral rehydration therapy. Lancet 1979;2:809-12.

Richmond JB. The needs of children. In: Knowles JH, ed. Doing better and feeling worse: health in the United States. New York: Norton, 1977:247-60.

Rohde JE, Northrop RS. Taking science where the diarrhea is. In: Acute diarrhea in childhood. Ciba Foundation Symposium 42 (new series). Amsterdam: Elsevier 1976:339-57.

Sack DA. Treatment of acute diarrhea with oral rehydration solution. Drugs 1982;23:150-57.

Santosham M, Dauron RS, Dillman L, et al. Oral rehydration therapy of infantile diarrhea. N Engl J Med 1982;306:1070-76.

Shirkey HC, ed. Pediatric therapy, 6th ed. St. Louis: Mosby, 1980:486.

Taylor B, Wadsworth J, Golding J, Butler N. Breast feeding, bronchitis, and admission for lower respiratory illness and gastroenteritis during the first five years. Lancet 1982;1:178-79.

USDHHS (U.S. Department of Health and Human Services). Public Health Service. National Center for Health Statistics. Vital statistics of the United States—1978. vol II—Mortality, part A. Hyattsville, Md.;1982.

Walker-Smith JA, Frischmann WJ, Khan S. Oral rehydration, diarrhea and general practice. Lancet 1983;1:178-79.

WHO (World Health Organization). Report of a field trial by an international study group, a positive effect on nutrition of Philippine children of an oral glucose-electrolyte solution given at home for the treatment of diarrhea. Bull WHO 1977;55:87–94.

Wittner M. Protozoan diarrhea. In: Lifshitz F, ed. Clinical disorders in pediatric gastroenterology and nutrition. New York: Dekker, 1980:229–48.

Woodward WE, Hirschhorn N, Sack RB, et al. Acute diarrhea on an Apache indian reservation. Am J Epidemiol 1974;99:281–90.

Part IV

Caveats, Considerations, and Conclusions

18
The Findings in Perspective

Barbara Starfield

This review unequivocally answers yes to the question, Does medical care make a difference? The evidence shows that the frequency of occurrence of conditions that can be prevented declines in response to the provision of medical care; that early detection, when it is appropriate, prevents the progression of conditions from the asymptomatic to the symptomatic state; and that indicated interventions reduce the occurrence of sequelae or prevent the condition from becoming serious. Furthermore, population groups in poorest health appear to benefit the most from improved access to medical care.

Nature of the Evidence

The basis for this conclusion was evidence of three types, two involving primarily population-based data and one involving primarily clinical data. In the first type, a theoretical reason to suspect a causal relationship between the provision of medical care and improved health, combined with changes in long-term trends in morbid events associated with a change in the health system, provided inferential evidence of benefit from medical care. Studies of this first type involved the collection of data on defined populations involving entire communities. Evidence for benefit of medical care was persuasive for reductions in neonatal and postneonatal mortality, prevention of adolescent childbearing, immunizations and consequent reductions in communicable diseases, prevention of complications of bacterial meningitis, diabetic ketoacidosis, rheumatic fever, and, in particular circumstances, in reducing the occurrence of low birth weight. The benefits of the vital statistics system are amply demonstrated by the usefulness of data on births and deaths, which are maintained by local jurisdictions as a matter of law, and which contain sociodemographic information that often facilitates understanding of the causes and correlates of morbid events. But these types of data are not available for most other health problems so that studies of this type are the exception rather than the rule. Data concerning the occurrence of most conditions in defined populations are scarce in societies characterized by fragmentation of services (and therefore fragmentation of information), as is the case in the United States.

The second type of evidence employing population-based data involved analysis of differences in severity of problems across different population groups. Although biologic or social factors might produce differences in the occurrence of illness, greater severity of illness is likely to be due more to lack of access to medical care, especially where efficacious regimens are available. This type of inferential evidence for benefit of medical care was found for neonatal mortality, bacterial meningitis, and diabetic ketoacidosis. In all three instances, the case was strengthened by data from clinical studies.

The major limitation of population-based data, from the viewpoint of contributing knowledge about the relationship between medical care and measures of ill health, is that the associations are ecological. That is, for the most part, analyses of the association between and among characteristics are at the ecological level. It requires a leap of faith to infer from relationships at the ecological level to relationships at the individual level. For example, the fact that the availability of abortions at the community level is associated with lower infant mortality does not necessarily prove that the individual deaths that were averted were a result of the seeking of an abortion, although the presumption is compelling. Concerns about possible invasion of privacy prevent the inclusion of much potentially identifying information on vital statistics records, and although efforts (for example, matched birth and death statistics and the National Death Index) can overcome some of these problems, most vital statistics records have limited usefulness as sources of information at the individual level. Findings from studies based upon vital statistics do, however, provide a good basis for hypotheses that can be tested by other types of data.

The third type of study used clinical data obtained in specific health facilities rather than population-based data from communities. In contrast to population-based data, clinical data can provide information about associations of characteristics at the individual level. Their major limitation lies in their unknown representativeness; it is always possible and often likely that the patients served and medical care provided in the facilities in which the studies are conducted are not the same as in the community at large. (See, for example, Ellenberg and Nelson 1980.) Moreover, whatever associations between characteristics are elucidated by clinical studies may not be representative of associations in other populations. Nevertheless, the consistency of findings from a variety of clinical studies conducted at different times, in different places, and by different investigators provides reasonable confidence in the conclusions. Studies using this type of evidence were predominant in the cases of appendicitis, asthma, epilepsy, gastroenteritis, child battering, and iron-deficiency anemia, and contributory in the cases of neonatal mortality, bacterial meningitis, and diabetes.

Summary of Evidence Regarding Specific Conditions

The nature of benefit where it was clearly evident varied with the condition under consideration. In the case of low birth weight, there was clear evidence of benefit from receipt of some prenatal care as compared with no prenatal care, and for early as compared with late receipt of care. However, benefit from increasing number of prenatal visits or from nutritional intervention was not completely persuasive, in the latter case primarily because study designs were not optimal. But there were notable successes in some specific instances. What characterized these is that they seemed to be primarily situations in which prenatal care was a part of ongoing care of the woman. If this is the case, it might be presumed that the reason for better outcome is attention before pregnancy to those conditions that are subsequently associated with poor outcome. It may be, for example, that the effects of poor nutrition and poor physical condition can be prevented only (or best) by interventions that antedate rather than accompany prenatal care.

Evidence of benefit in the prevention of neonatal mortality was convincing, although some of it was indirect. To the extent that medical care was targeted at disadvantaged populations, as was the case with organized family planning activities, Medicaid as a source of payment, and (where available) abortions, it reduced the disparity between disadvantaged and nondisadvantaged populations. Neonatal intensive care, while not subjected to controlled clinical trial (except in one instance) seems to have had a major impact in reducing mortality and morbidity; regionalization of services to facilitate access to such care has been effective. Curiously, and despite the benefit derived from neonatal intensive care, the gap in neonatal mortality rates between the poor and the nonpoor has not narrowed. Perhaps this is because this technological development, in contrast to the other types of interventions, is not targeted specifically at reducing disparities among different population groups. There is, for example, evidence that at least one "technology," amniocentesis, has been relatively more available to the well-off than to the disadvantaged (Powledge 1976; Sokal et al. 1980; Bannerman et al. 1977). It is possible, however, that one of the benefits of Medicaid has been its facilitation of access to neonatal intensive care, and the differences among states in the availability of financing by Medicaid of prenatal services (Davidson 1980) may account for the absence of a systemwide effect of intensive care in reducing the poor–nonpoor gap. The same could be postulated regarding the beneficial effects of prenatal care and community clinics, which are not uniformly distributed across the country. Indirect evidence of benefit from targeting resources is provided by an analysis of mortality rates and standardized mortality ratios in the health services areas of the United States. In this study (Foster and Kleinman 1982), expected neonatal mortality rates were calculated by applying standard birth weight–specific neonatal mortality rates to the birth weight distributions of each area's births. A standardized mortality ratio was calculated for each area by dividing the observed neonatal mortality rate by the expected neonatal mortality rate. The data from this analysis suggest that geographic variation in neonatal mortality among the HSAs in the United States is due more to variations in weight-specific mortality than to variations in birth weight distribution. Comparison of the standardized crude neonatal mortality ratios in those areas with higher than expected neonatal mortality rates showed that there were some areas that did not have high standardized mortality despite their relatively high mortality rates. In these areas, the presumption was that targeting of medical care resources where they were most needed was responsible for their lower than expected mortality. Evidence of the impact of targeting is also provided by data from income-maintenance studies, although in these studies the outcome variable was birth weight rather than mortality and the intervention was income rather than medical care. In one study (Kehrer and Wolin 1979) exposure to income supplements was specifically beneficial to infants born to mothers at high risk. However, the effect was not related to receipt of prenatal care, and supplemental exploratory investigation suggested that general improvement in nutrition may have been part of the causal chain. However, a subsequent study of income maintenance (Kehrer and Wolin 1980) failed to confirm the earlier results. Significantly, neither experiment included consideration of the presence of insurance or Medicaid eligibility and their differential impacts on families at varying risk.

The mechanism for the significant beneficial impact of abortion on neonatal mortality is difficult to document. High-risk characteristics are much more common among women with abortions than those having live births. In 1980, 0.3 percent of mothers of live births were under age 15, and 15.3 percent were 15–19; the comparable percentages for women undergoing abortion were 1 percent and 28.2 percent. More than three quarters (76.7 percent) of women undergoing abortion were unmarried as compared with 18.9 percent among mothers of live-born infants. It is likely that abortion preferentially reduces births to high-risk women, thus indirectly resulting in lower mortality rates, especially neonatal mortality rates. Review of the data on teenage childbearing showed that where abortion is available, births to this high-risk population are reduced. Declines in neonatal mortality, even in areas in which they were associated in time with the legalization of abortion, were birth weight specific (Pakter and Nelson 1974); this, and the evidence that the availability of abortions reduces the likelihood of low birth weight (especially very low birth weight) suggest that abortions reduce births at high risk rather than reducing the mortality of infants born at high risk. Being born out of wedlock is also a risk factor affected by abortion. Infant mortality rates have always been higher for infants born out of wedlock than for those born in wedlock (NCHS 1980) even after the availability of abortions (Pakter and Nelson 1974). In New York City, the percentage decrease in number of births after legalization of abortion was greater for out-of-wedlock than for in-wedlock births, especially among whites. A mother's inability to obtain an abortion may increase her infant's chance of a poor outcome, perhaps as a result of failure of the mother to seek optimal medical care for an unwanted pregnancy. If failure to receive optimal prenatal care were the medical care factor responsible for the effect, then controlling for receipt of prenatal care should reduce the effect of marital status. However, later exposure to prenatal care does not appear to be the explanatory factor, as the differentials in mortality by marital status are greatest when prenatal care is received early in pregnancy (NCHS 1980).

Examination of changes in the cause of infant mortality (including both neonatal and postneonatal components) in two time periods, one before and one after the availability of abortions, suggest that the effectiveness of abortions may be, in part, a result of the subsequent decrease in births of unwanted children. Data obtained from 50 states in 1971–72 and 1974–75 show significant decreases in rates of infant mortality from nonvehicle accidental deaths, and the effect was most marked in states where there were fewest abortions before the Supreme Court decision and where increases in abortion occurred following the decision. Many nonvehicle accidental deaths are associated with situations characterized by prolonged parental inattention. No other cause of death (with the possible exception of homicide) changed in frequency between the two time periods (Robertson 1981). Thus it appears likely that whereas the impact of abortion in reducing neonatal mortality is primarily associated with reductions in high-risk births, the effect of being unwanted is more related to reductions in postneonatal mortality.

The excess of postneonatal mortality in the United States as compared with other industrialized nations is due to deaths from accidents and infectious diseases, not congenital causes. Evidence, while not abundant, is persuasive in showing that deaths in the first year of life past the period shortly after birth are amenable to prevention by both social and medical interventions. Income maintenance is associated with a significant decrease in the proportion of deaths that are postneonatal (and without an increase in the total number of deaths) (Kehrer and Wolin 1980). Both the presence of community health centers and greater expenditures for medical care are ecologically associated with lower postneonatal mortality rates, and the effect of the latter on postneonatal mortality is greater than its effect on neonatal mortality.

Benefit of medical care was also suggested by population-based studies concerning births to teenage mothers, communicable diseases, and acute rheumatic fever. For births to teenage mothers, there was convincing evidence of the benefit of abortions in particular, and for family planning in general.

For communicable disease, data from the Centers for Disease Control showed that immunization rates and communicable disease rates follow closely the input of resources to support immunization programs. It is of particular interest that these conclusions differ from those of other authors who have examined long-term trends in death rates for a variety of diseases (e.g., diphtheria, pertussis, poliomyelitis, measles) and have concluded that the introduction of technologies such as immunization have had little impact (Kass 1971; McKinlay and McKinlay 1977). Several factors account for the discrepancies. First, the analyses of these investigators have been limited to mortality data. Second, over very long periods of time (i.e., many decades to a century), it is likely that the benefits of medical care were dwarfed by more pervasive social and environmental changes, as occurred in the developed countries in which the studies were done. Third (and most relevant to the central focus of this book) is the fact that these studies have examined only the relationship between the development of particular technologies and their impact, not the means and adequacy of their application. The evidence produced in the chapter on immunizations and communicable diseases (as well as in other chapters) makes it clear that the existence of a technology is not sufficient for benefit to be derived from it. This evidence should be persuasive in arguing for much more attention to issues concerning the optimum methods of health services delivery.

For rheumatic fever, comprehensive care programs, which facilitated the appropriate use of diagnostic techniques and therapy, were associated with reductions in frequency of both initial and recurrent attacks. It was not clear that all of the decline in incidence rates was attributable to medical care, as it began before the era of efficacious medical prophylaxis.

In the cases of bacterial meningitis and diabetic ketoacidosis, the availability of both population-based and clinical data contributed to an understanding of the relationship between access to medical care and its impact. In both cases, the availability of the two different types of evidence strengthened the conclusion that access to medical care reduces the occurrence or likelihood of adverse effect of the condition. Population-based data made it possible to compare the frequency of occurrence of bacterial meningitis in geographic areas differing in sociodemographic characteristics that were known to differ in access to medical care. Clinical data documented the relationship between delay in receipt of care and the occurrence of sequelae. Both types of studies provided convincing evidence that relatively poor access to medical care is associated with an increased likelihood of a poorer prognosis from the illness. The availability of both types of evidence in the case of diabetic ketoacidosis also facilitated conclusions about the benefits of medical care, although there were many fewer studies than was the case for meningitis. Population-based studies documented the greater likelihood of occurrence of this preventable complication of diabetes in poor children, and clinical studies showed reductions in hospitalizations consequent to improvements in access to care.

For the remainder of the conditions, the available evidence was only of the clinical type. Studies from at least seven different hospitals indicated that delay in seeking care was associated with increased likelihood of complications from appendicitis; these and the studies showing increased rates of complications in individuals at socioeconomic disadvantage provided dependable evidence for the beneficial impact of access to medical care.

Few studies examined the effectiveness of medical care for asthma, despite its high frequency. Both deaths and hospitalizations appear to be reduced when there is a continuous source of care available to the individual with asthma. Although most of the studies were hardly models of exemplary research design, they did suggest that both hospitalization and deaths are preventable at least some the of the time with good ongoing care.

The challenge to medical care for the prevention of congenital hypothyroidism and phenylketonuria concerns the organization of services at a community level rather than the efficacy of medical diagnosis and management, which are well established. These conditions can be prevented with standard medical care, but the rapidity and accuracy of diagnosis greatly influence the outcome of medical management. There is at least suggestive evidence that the availability of centralized laboratories that perform the diagnostic tests is important in early diagnosis. Centralization greatly enhances quality control; increased decentralization of laboratories is likely to be associated with an increase in the frequency of missed or delayed diagnoses.

For child battering, evidence of the benefits of medical care interventions was mixed. However, the weight of current evidence suggests that certain types of attention in the perinatal period lessen the likelihood of abuse in families at high risk.

There is some doubt about the contribution of medical care only with regard to 2 of the 16 reviewed conditions. For iron-deficiency anemia, the evidence was fragmentary and based primarily on isolated demonstration programs. Part of the problem with this condition may be the lack of consensus on the significance of milder degrees of anemia and the general lack of recognition of the condition except where there is routine screening for it.

Deaths and encephalopathy resulting from lead poisoning now occur only rarely. This progress was undoubtedly a result of many changes of the 1960s and 1970s, including the development of an efficacious method of reducing body burdens of lead and greatly increased access to medical care that undoubtedly facilitated the earlier diagnosis and treatment of toxicity. However, it is clear that there have been a variety of factors responsible for the enormous decline in occurrence of acute toxicity from lead, including reduction in lead in gasoline and paint, imposition of standards for industrial emissions, and possibly the lead paint prevention program. Despite the near-disappearance of acute lead toxicity in children, levels of lead just under the acute toxicity threshold are a continuing problem in many communities, with probable consequences for impairment of cognition and behavior in children with the elevations.

For the remaining two conditions, epilepsy and gastroenteritis, the evidence bearing on the issue of effectiveness was sparse. For epilepsy, there was suggestive evidence that good ongoing care reduces the likelihood of seizures and facilitates psychosocial adaptation to the condition. For gastroenteritis, there was clear evidence of the efficacy of oral rehydration solutions for prevention of hospitalization, and at least suggestive evidence of the importance of access to medical care in preventing untoward sequelae.

The Context of the Findings

This relatively charitable view of the benefits of medical care is consistent with the conclusions drawn by other observers of the medical care scene. A recent review of the benefits of well-child care concluded that medical care is generally beneficial, although the nature of the evidence was different from that used in this monograph (Shadish 1982). Blendon and Rogers (1983) referred to a number of instances where measures of health were remarkably improved coincident with better access to better medical care. From 1968 to 1980, the expectation of life at birth increased four years, adjusted death rates dropped by 20 percent, and there were reductions in deaths from 10 of the 15 leading killers. McDermott and colleagues (1972) documented the effect of personal health care in reducing the sequelae of otitis media under conditions where social disadvantage seriously compromised the overall effectiveness of medical care. Inman (1976), in an analysis of data from a community-based study in Washington, D.C., showed that an increase in income or health insurance improved child health as measured by the reduced occurrence of otitis media. Although the effect was small (on the order of 1–3 percent), the value of doctor visits in public facilities for families with low maternal education was an important predictor of better health. There is evidence of overall benefit as a result of improved access to care in the mid-1960s (Starfield 1982) and documentation of the beneficial impact from a variety of specific programs resulting from governmental support of health programs to improve access to care in needy areas. A study of the Medicaid EPSDT (Early and Periodic Screening, Detection, and Treatment) program in Pennsylvania (Irwin and Conroy-Hughes 1982) showed that periodic screening under the program was associated with a decrease in the prevalence of abnormalities requiring care. Studies at specific sites where there were Maternity and Infant Care projects showed reduced maternal morbidity, stillbirth rates, number of premature infants, neonatal mortality, and infant mortality (Davis and Schoen 1978). Komaroff and Duffel (1976) implied a possible causal relationship between the presence of an M & I project and decreased neonatal mortality. A 1975 survey of almost 21,000 individuals at five urban community health centers (CHCs) provided evidence that CHCs contribute to lower utilization of hospital services than other delivery forms (Freeman and Goetsch 1980). Regression analyses holding constant the effects of age, sex, race, income, education, and health status found hospital admission rates 50 percent lower for CHC patients than for patients in hospital outpatient departments and 30 percent lower than for patients who receive care from private physicians (Davis 1982). A study of individuals eligible for Medicaid who received care from CHCs had fewer hospital admissions and fewer total hospital days than other Medicaid recipients. Earlier studies by Klein et al. (1973), Zwick (1972), and Bellin et al. (1969) also demonstrated that CHCs reduce hospitalization. These beneficial effects of CHCs may be a result of their special organizational features as well as their greater accessibility. As Rogers, Blendon, and Moloney (1982) point out, a direct causal relationship between availability of medical care and improved health cannot be inferred from most of these studies, but the consistency of the findings and the logic of the association is compelling.

What explains the discrepancy between these charitable views of the benefits of medical care and the views of those who doubt that medical care has much to offer (Carlson 1975; Illich 1976; McKeown 1979; McKinlay and McKinlay 1977)? While it is clear that medical care can and does make a difference, it is equally clear that some declines in the occurrence of illness over time have resulted from social changes rather than from improvements in access to medical care or in the content of medical care, even for some of the conditions discussed in this book. For example, declines in the rate of infant mortality in the early decades of the twentieth century were largely a result of declines in the incidence of infectious diseases and advances in nutrition that came about as a response to improvements in sanitation and the provision of infant food by public and private agencies at the local level (Cheney 1984). In the long term, the effect of medical care is dominated by concomitant and stronger advances in the social realm. Medical care efforts, which occur at the margin, become invisible when viewed against the larger picture. Moreover, these more global analyses capture only phenomena for which there are available data; in the main these consist of mortality statistics. Postponement of death is but one function of medical care; equally noble functions are prevention of illness, alleviation of disturbing manifestations of illness, and interruption of the progression of illness.

In many ways, medical care is a prisoner of a nomenclature that makes it difficult to demonstrate these aspects of its usefulness. Existing systems of classification are based primarily on causes of death or on biophysical derangements. The International Classification of Diseases (ICD) was developed and is useful for coding problems associated with death, but is much less useful for coding morbidity. Despite this, most reimbursement systems require a diagnosis listed in the ICD or its adaptations, even though most of medical care consists of the management of problems that cannot be classified as an ICD diagnosis. Moreover, abnormalities that are manifested by a numerical laboratory result can be more readily used for research and patient care than behavioral or functional abnormalities for which there are still no standardized classifications (McDermott 1981). Approaches to dealing with this situation have been suggested (McDermott 1981; Starfield 1974; Ware et al. 1981) but none have yet been implemented on a wide scale. However, new developments in terminology that make it possible to specify the variety of morbidity as it presents in nonhospital practice (WONCA 1979; Schneider 1979) and new methods for classifying physical and behavioral functioning (see, for example, Stein and Jessop 1982; Eisen et al. 1979) will probably facilitate demonstration of the effects of medical care, both in general and with regard to population groups with greatest need for it.

The limitations of the approach used in this review should not be minimized. Fewer than a handful of the cited studies were controlled trials, and none were conducted using double-blind methods of allocating subjects to study groups. In this regard, however, the studies are not atypical of the medical literature in general including those studies that provide the basis for most clinical decision making (Glantz 1980; Sheehan 1980; Williamson et al. 1979; Chalmers et al. 1983; Diamond and Forrester 1983). Fortunately, some of the studies included special types of analyses so that there is confidence in the conclusions despite the limitations. The major source of confidence, however, lies in the replicability of the findings from many studies done at different times by different investigators and in different locales. It is true, however, that the conclusions reached from this review might not be generalizable to medical care for the conditions that were not included. The conditions were chosen at least in part because medical care "experts" believed them to be particularly susceptible to medical care interventions, and because there was likely to be a literature that supported this conclusion. Some conditions were eliminated from consideration because they did not fulfill these criteria, even though there were studies that examined the efficacy of particular modes of therapy for them.

Challenges for the Future

The need to demonstrate benefit from medical care is not something that has always been a priority. In many countries there is no imperative to do so, even while large amounts of public funds are spent to provide, free of charge, basic services to mothers and children on the assumption that this will produce an overall benefit to society. In the United States rapidly increasing costs, due in large measure to the absence of a mechanism for setting priorities for care and the continuing explosion in availability and use of medical technology, engenders pressure from both private and public payors to be more selective in the reimbursement of medical care procedures. As a result, there is increasing interest in evaluation before a procedure is widely adopted. As yet, however, there is little translation of this interest to financial or organizational support for the kinds of studies that are required. Demonstrations of efficacy, in which the impact of a technology or other intervention is determined under controlled conditions, are properly under the jurisdiction of an agency such as the National Institutes of Health, which has a long history of excellence in biomedical and clinical research. Once efficacy is demonstrated, there remains the challenge of the appropriate and adequate distribution of the technology or intervention. Studies of the usefulness of an intervention when applied in the general population, in the absence of control over its use, require a different set of skills and different types of data than are employed in studies of efficacy. Demonstration of effectiveness, cost-effectiveness, and equity require multidisciplinary perspectives and techniques, and data systems that can provide denominators (populations at risk) as well as numerators (populations reached by the intervention) for their conduct. At present, interest in these types of studies is scattered throughout the public and private sectors, but responsibility is located in a variety of federal agencies that have no clear mandate to carry out the function and no defined budget for the specific purpose. Even the National Center for Health Services Research, the federal agency most nearly suited to bear the responsibility, suffered severe cuts in its budget over the decade of the seventies. The private sector shows little inclination to take up the slack. For example, only .06 percent of total domestic health giving by foundations is directed at national and community statistics that provide the denominators for the needed studies. Less than 4 percent of all foundation dollars spent on health are targeted at health services research, the discipline that deals with the subjects of effectiveness, efficacy, and costs (Dooley et al. 1983). A serious attempt to determine whether and under what circumstances medical care makes a difference will require a more focused approach than has been the case in the past. There is little doubt that the requirement for accountability in the expenditure of funds will increase in priority. The commitment of public monies for medical care is not likely to be reversed, and the burgeoning of new technologies is not likely to abate. There seems little chance for continuation of the laissez-faire approach to medical care that has characterized the past, and there are not many alternatives that will be acceptable to the profession. Even more rigid control over the dispensation of technology as is inevitable with attempts to "corporatize" medical care delivery, will require better information about the usefulness of various aspects of medical practice. Although some attempts to cap health expenditures, limit clearly redundant utilization, regulate fees and physician supply, and change reimbursement mechanisms will clearly be needed (Platt 1983), it will not be possible to incorporate rationality into the process of decision making without information about the benefits of specific interventions. From the point of view of society overall, it is the small but very frequent technologies—those that comprise much of the office-based practice of medicine—that contribute most to the rapidly increasing costs of care (Moloney and Rogers 1979). It is therefore in office-based practice that we must look for the evidence that they are useful. Perhaps more than ever before it seems opportune for the profession to devise its own approaches to encouraging responsible technologic innovation and medical creativity. Building a mechanism for the conduct of clinical trials of new and existing interventions is an important component of this strategy, but it is useful primarily in the long run. In the meantime, there are decisions to be made about the dispensation of medical care, and there is danger that those who are dependent upon society's help in attaining it will be deprived under the guise of "no demonstrable evidence of benefit." Two major statements of national policy, one in the United States and one in Canada, appear to have been heavily influenced in their recommendation by this perceived lack of evidence of benefit. In contrast, this review suggests that those who are most in need of medical care may have the most to gain from better access to it. Access alone seems to be associated with benefit, perhaps at least in part by what has been called the Samaritan function of medical care, that is, that function that provides compassion and reassurance rather than the application of some mechanical technology (McDermott 1978). The review also suggests that a combination of population-based and clinical approaches to data collection will be required to demonstrate the benefits of medical care. Population-based research provides the hypotheses for clinical research, and it provides the denominators that make it possible to interpret events in their broad context (Starfield 1981).

What should be the basis of society's decisions about the allocation of services? The time has come for clinical practitioners, public health professionals, and academic researchers to take on a new and joint role in public policy formation. Heretofore absent from the process that documents health needs, health processes, and the results of health care, practitioners must now begin to work with academicians and public health colleagues to determine the type and magnitude of health problems in their communities, discover geographic areas where frequencies of occurrence of problems are relatively high, develop plans for meeting those needs, and document improvements consequent to the provision of care. There is already recognition among some segments of the professional community of the need to build a research base within the practice of medicine instead of peripheral to it as has been the case in the past. New data systems are being developed to facilitate the process of collaboration in the design and conduct of research into important questions of effectiveness of care, and there is excitement associated with the realization that the practice of medicine can be a source of new knowledge for the advancement of the science and art of medical care (Nelson et al. 1981; Green et al. 1983). The benefits of medical care cannot be determined in the traditional laboratory; the concept of "the laboratory" needs to be broadened to encompass the community.

Major investment in new approaches to evaluation will not come easily. But, after all, it is the noblest of society's goals—better health of its people—that is at issue.

References

Bannerman R, Gillick D, Van Coevering R, Knobloch N, Ingall G. Amniocentesis and educational attainment. N Engl J Med 1977; 297:449.

Bellin S, Geiger J, Gibson C. Impact of ambulatory health care services on the demand for hospital beds. N Engl J Med 1969;280:808–12.

Blendon R, Rogers D. Cutting medical care costs. JAMA 1983;250:1880–85.

Carlson R. The end of medicine. New York: John Wiley & Sons, 1975.

Chalmers T, Celano P, Sacks H, Smith H. Bias in treatment assignment in controlled clinical trials. N Engl J Med 1983; 309:1358–61.

Cheney R. Seasonal aspects of infant and childhood mortality: Philadelphia, 1865–1920. J Interdis Hist 1984;14;561–85.

Davidson S. Medicaid decisions: a systematic analysis of the cost problems. Cambridge, Mass.: Bollinger, 1980.

Davis K. Contracting with community health centers. In: Blendon R, Moloney T, eds. New approaches to the Medicaid crisis. New York: Frost and Sullivan, 1982:199–217.

Davis K, Schoen C. Health and the war on poverty: A ten-year appraisal. Washington, D.C.: Brookings Institution, 1978.

Diamond G, Forrester J. Clinical trials and statistical verdicts: probable grounds for appeal. Ann Intern Med 1983;98:385–94.

Dooley B, Jackson C, Merrill J, Reuter J, Tyson K. DataWatch: how do private foundations spend their money. Health Aff 1983;2:104–14.

Eisen M, Ware J, Donald C, Brook R. Measuring components of children's health. Med Care 1979;17:902–21.

Ellenberg J, Nelson K. Sample selection and the natural history of disease: studies of febrile seizures. JAMA 1980;243:1337–40.

Foster JE, Kleinman JC. Adjusting national mortality rates for birth weight. NCHS. Vital health stat, series 2, no. 94, 1982 (DHHS publication no. (PHS)82-1368).

Freeman H, Goetsch G. Use of community health centers: summary tables. Los Angeles: Institute for Social Science Research, University of California, 1980:1–60.

Glantz S. Biostatistics: how to detect, correct, and prevent errors in the medical literature. Circulation 1980;61:1–7.

Green L, Wood M, Becker L, et al. The ambulatory sentinel practice network: purpose, method, and policies. Unpublished manuscript, 1983.

Illich I. Medical nemesis: the expropriation of health. New York: Pantheon Books, 1976.

Inman R. The family provision of children's health: an economic analysis. In: Rosett R, ed. The role of health insurance in the health services sector. New York: Neale Watson Academic Publications for the National Bureau of Economic Research, 1976.

Irwin P, Conroy-Hughes R. EPSDT impact on health status: estimates based on secondary analysis of administratively-generated data. Med Care 1982;10:216–34.

Kass E. Infectious disease and social change. J Infect Dis 1971;123:110–14.

Kehrer B, Wolin C. Impact of income maintenance on low birth weight: evidence from the Gary experiment. J Hum Resour 1979;14:434-62.

Kehrer B, Wolin C. Impact of the Seattle-Denver income maintenance experiment on adverse pregnancy outcomes. Princeton, N.J.: Mathematics Policy Research, 1980.

Klein M, Roghmann K, Woodward K, Charney E. The impact of Rochester neighborhood health centers on hospitalization of children, 1968-1970. Pediatrics 1973;51:833-39.

Komaroff A, Duffel B. An evaluation of selected federal categorical health programs for the poor. Am J Public Health 1976;66:255-61.

McDermott W. Medicine: the public good and one's own. Persp Biol Med 1978;21:167-87.

McDermott W. Absence of indicators of the influence of its physicians on a society's health. Am J Med 1981;70:833-43.

McDermott W, Deuschle K, Barnett C. Health care experiment at many farms. Science 1972;175:23-31.

McKeown T. The role of medicine: dream, mirage, or nemesis? Princeton, N.J.: Princeton University Press, 1979.

McKinlay J, McKinlay S. The questionable contribution of medical measures to the decline of mortality of the United States in the twentieth century. Milbank Mem Fund Q/ Health & Society 1977;55:405-28.

Moloney T, Rogers D. Medical technology—a different view of the contentious debate over costs. N Engl J Med 1979;301:1413-19.

NCHS (National Center for Health Statistics). Factors associated with low birth weight, U.S., 1976. Vital Health Stat, series 21, no. 37, 1980 (DHEW publication no. (PHS)80-1915).

Nelson E, Kirk J, Bise B, et al. The cooperative information project: part 1: a sentinel practice network for service and research in primary care. J Fam Pract 1981;13:641-49.

Pakter J, Nelson F. Factors in the unprecedented decline in infant mortality in New York City. Bull NY Acad Med 1974;50:839-68.

Platt R. Cost-containment—another view. N Engl J Med 1983;309:726-30.

Powledge T. Prenatal diagnosis—now the problems. New Scientist 1976; 69:332-34.

Robertson L. Abortion and infant mortality before and after the 1973 U.S. Supreme Court decision on abortion. J Biosoc Sci 1981;13:275-80.

Rogers D, Blendon R, Moloney T. Who needs Medicaid? N Engl J Med 1982;307:13-18.

Schneider D. A reason for visit classification for ambulatory care. NCHS. Vital health stat, series 2, no. 78, February 1979 (DHEW publication no. (PHS)79-1352).

Shadish W. A review and critique of controlled studies of the effectiveness of preventive child health care. Health Policy Q 1982;2:24-52.

Sheehan T. The medical literature: let the researchers beware. Arch Intern Med 1980;140:472-74.

Sokal DC, Byrd JR, Chen ATL, Goldberg MF, Oakley GP. Prenatal chromosomal diagnosis: racial and geographic variation for older women in Georgia. JAMA 1980;244:1355–57.

Starfield B. Measurement of outcome: a proposed scheme. Milbank Mem Fund Q 1974;52:39–50.

Starfield B. Patients and populations: necessary links between the two approaches to pediatric research. Pediatr Res 1981;15:1–5.

Starfield B. Family income, ill health, and medical care of U.S. children. J Public Health Policy 1982;3:244–59.

Stein R, Jessop D. A noncategorical approach to chronic childhood illness. Public Health Rep 1982;97:354–62.

Ware J, Brook R, Davies A, Lohr K. Choosing measures of health status for individuals in general populations. Am J Public Health 1981;71:620–25.

Williamson J, Goldschmidt P, Jillson I. Medical practice information demonstration project: Final report, 1979 (Contract 282-77-0068GS, Office of the Assistant Secretary for Health, DHEW).

WONCA (World Organization of National Colleges, Academies and Academic Associations of General Practitioners/Family Physicians). International classification of health problems in primary care. Oxford: Oxford University Press, 1979.

Zwick D. Some accomplishments and findings of neighborhood health centers. Milbank Mem Fund Q 1972;50 (pt. 2):387–421.

Notes on Contributors

BARBARA STARFIELD, M.D., M.P.H., a pediatrician, epidemiologist, and public health professional, has a major commitment to the improvement of health care for the population. Her contributions include the development of methods for measuring various aspects of the health care system, primary care, and outcome of care. Her current research addresses psychosocial problems in childhood and issues related to the impact of public policy on health care and health status, both nationally and internationally. She directs the Division of Health Policy at the Johns Hopkins University School of Hygiene and Public Health. At the time this book was written, she was a Henry J. Kaiser Senior Fellow at the Center for Advanced Study in the Behavioral Sciences.

LISA EGBUONU, M.D., M.P.H., received her degrees in a joint program from the Johns Hopkins University School of Medicine and the School of Hygiene and Public Health. Currently a second-year pediatric resident at the Children's Hospital of Philadelphia, she plans to pursue a career in public health planning and policy with particular emphasis on issues affecting children's health.

MARK FARFEL is a doctoral candidate in the Department of Health Policy and Management of the Johns Hopkins University School of Hygiene and Public Health. He is currently conducting a randomized control trial of alternative methods for reducing household lead exposure among children in a project supported in part by the National Center for Health Services Research.

NANCY HUTTON, M.D., is a member of the faculty in the Division of Primary Care and Adolescent Medicine at the Johns Hopkins University School of Medicine. Her interests include assessing the effectiveness of common pediatric practices and the primary care of children with chronic problems.

ALAIN JOFFE, M.D., M.P.H., is assistant professor of pediatrics at the Johns Hopkins University School of Medicine and director of the Adolescent Medicine Program there. His major areas of interest and research include sexually transmitted diseases, psychosomatic illness, and the application of quantitative methods to defining and teaching "clinical judgment."

LAWRENCE S. WISSOW, M.D., is the Child Health Specialist for the Office of the Secretary, Maryland Department of Health and Mental Hygiene. He is also a member of the faculty in pediatrics at the Johns Hopkins University School of Medicine.

Index

Abortion, 40–41, 42–44
    impact of, on teenage fertility, 43–44, 149
    and low birth weight, 29–30, 148
    and neonatal mortality, 13–15, 17, 147, 148–49
    and socioeconomic differentials, 43
Abuse, child. *See* Child abuse
Access to care, 91–92, 151, 152–53, 156
    for abortions, 44
    for appendicitis, 126, 128
    for asthma, 131
    for bacterial meningitis, 112–13, 115–17
    for diabetes, 99–101
    for epilepsy, 107
    for gastroenteritis, 138
    for prenatal care, 30–31
Accidental deaths, 149
Air pollution, 131. *See also* Environment, lead in
Amniocentesis, availability of, 147
Anemia, iron-deficiency, 87–93, 151
Antibiotics
    in bacterial meningitis, 112–13, 116
    in diabetes, 99
    inappropriate use of, in asthma, 132
    in prevention of rheumatic fever, 59, 60
Appendicitis, 120–28, 146, 150
Asthma, 130–33, 146, 151
Availability of services, 107. *See also* Access to care; Medical expenditures, public; Physicians

Bacterial meningitis, 109–17, 145, 146, 150
Births, out-of-wedlock. *See* Illegitimacy

Birth weight, and infant mortality, 9, 16. *See also* Low birth weight
Birth weight–specific mortality, 16, 22, 147, 148

Case fatality
    in appendicitis, 120
    in bacterial meningitis, 109, 112–13, 116–17
    in gastroenteritis, 136, 138
    in pertussis, 53
Cause of death, 149
    in postneonatal period, 20–21
Centralization of facilities, 72–74, 151
Child abuse (battering), 63–67, 146, 151
Classification
    of disease, 153–54
    of morbidity, 153–54
Clinical studies, 3–4, 146, 150–51, 155–56
Clinical trials
    controlled, xv, 4, 16, 154
    regarding child battering, 64
    regarding iron-deficiency anemia, 92
Communicable disease, 48–56
Community-based studies, importance of, 3, 145–46, 149–50, 155–56
Community health centers, 17, 22, 147, 149, 152–53
Comprehensive care, 31, 32–33, 43, 54, 61, 147, 150
Congenital conditions, legislation regarding, 73
Consent, parental, 40–41
Continuity of care, 33, 54, 132, 147, 151, 152
Contraception, 40, 41–42
Cost effectiveness, 60, 82, 100, 138

Costs of care, 1, 155
   in diabetes, 98–99
   for screening, 73

Day care
   gastroenteritis in, 137, 138
   immunizations in, 56
   meningitis in, 112
Deaths. *See* Mortality
Delay in receipt of care, 150–51. *See also* Diagnosis
   for abortions, 44
   for appendicitis, 122, 126–28
   for asthma, 133
   for bacterial meningitis, 113–16
   for congenital conditions, 71, 72–73, 74
Diabetes, 97–101, 145, 146, 150
Diagnosis
   changing criteria for, in lead poisoning, 77
   decentralization of facilities and, 74
   importance of
      in appendicitis, 122, 126, 128
      in asthma, 132
      in bacterial meningitis, 114, 116–17
      in diabetes, 97
      in epilepsy, 107
      in lead poisoning, 78, 151
Diet, in phenylketonuria, 71–72. *See also* Nutrition
Diphtheria, 48
Disadvantaged populations
   reductions in risk to, 139, 145, 147, 148, 151, 152
   regarding low birth weight, 24, 33
   regarding neonatal mortality, 12, 15, 17
   regarding post neonatal mortality, 21–22
   regarding teenage pregnancy, 43
Diseases, International Classification of, 153
Disparities, racial. *See* Race, disparities associated with
Disparities, socioeconomic. *See* Income, low
Drugs. *See* Medication

Education, health. *See* Health education
Effectiveness, definition and measurement of, xv–xvi, 2–3, 4, 60, 155, 156. *See also sections of individual chapters*
Efficacy, xv–xvi, 3, 4, 150. *See also sections of individual chapters*
   of antibiotics in preventing rheumatic fever, 59
   of diet for preventing phenylketonuria, 71
   for iron-deficiency anemia, 87, 90–91
   of treatment for congenital hypothyroidism, 71
Environment, lead in, 77
Epidemiologic studies, 3, 16. *See also* Population-based studies
Epilepsy, 103–7, 146, 151–52
EPSDT (Early and Periodic Screening, Detection, and Treatment), 81, 92, 152
Expenditures. *See* Medical expenditures, public

Family planning, 13–15, 17, 40, 41–42, 44, 147, 149
Fatality. *See* Case fatality
Federal programs, impact of, 2, 113. *See also* Community health centers; EPSDT; Hyde Amendment; Lead Paint Poisoning Prevention Program; Legislation; Maternity and Infant Care; Medicaid; WIC
   on lead poisoning, 80–82
   on low birth weight, 26–29, 30–32
   on measles incidence, 54–56
   on immunizations, 54–55
   on infant mortality, 10–11
   on postneonatal mortality, 20
Financing. *See* Federal programs, impact of; Insurance, impact of; Legislation; State programs, for diagnostic testing
Fluid therapy, 137–38, 152
Foster care, 66

Gastroenteritis, 136–39, 146, 151–52
  in day care, 137, 138
  in migrant workers, 137
  on Indian reservations, 137
  oral rehydration for, 137–38, 152
German measles. *See* Rubella
Gestation age, 16, 24, 28–29, 31, 32
  and abortions, 41, 44
Group practice, prepaid, 12, 13, 132
  and prenatal care, 32–33
Governmental programs. *See* Federal programs, impact of; Legislation; Regulation relating to lead poisoning; State programs, for diagnostic testing

Health Centers. *See* Community health centers
Health education
  for asthma, 133
  for gastroenteritis, 137
  in prenatal care, 31
  for teenagers, 41
Health insurance. *See* Insurance, impact of
Health services research, 155
HMOs (health maintenance organizations). *See* Group practice, prepaid
Hospitalization, 152–53
  in asthma, 130, 132, 151
  in child battering, 64–65
  delay in, for appendicitis, 122, 126
  in diabetes, 98–99, 100, 101
  in gastroenteritis, 136, 152
  in pertussis, 53
  in rheumatic fever, 60–61
Hyde Amendment, 44
Hypothyroidism, congenital, 71–74, 151

Illegitimacy, 37, 38, 39, 148–49
Immunization Initiative, 48, 54–55
Immunizations, 48–56, 145, 149–50
  in preschoolers, 50–51
  in teenagers, 51–52, 53, 56
Incidence, 4. *See also sections in individual chapters*

Income, low. *See also* Disadvantaged populations
  and access to care, 43, 139
  and health
    in appendicitis, 127
    in asthma, 130
    in bacterial meningitis, 110, 116
    in diabetes, 97–98
    in epilepsy, 103
    in iron-deficiency anemia, 89–90
    in lead poisoning, 76
    in low birth weight, 24, 33
    in neonatal mortality, 17
    in postneonatal mortality, 22
    in rheumatic fever, 58, 62
  and immunization rates, 51
Income maintenance, 148, 149
Infant mortality. *See* Mortality, infant
Insurance, impact of, 152
  in diabetes, 99
  in gastroenteritis, 138
  in teenage pregnancies, 39
International Classification of Diseases, 153
Intrauterine growth retardation, 24, 31
  in rubella, 53
Iron-deficiency anemia, 87–93, 146, 151

Ketoacidosis, diabetic, 98, 99, 100, 145, 146
Knowledge, importance of. *See also* Health education
  about asthma, 132–33
  about epilepsy, 107
  about iron-deficiency anemia, 92–93
  concerning medication, 132

Laboratories for diagnostic testing, 72–74
Lead
  in air, 77, 82
  in dust, 78, 81
  in food, 82
  in gasoline, 77, 82, 151
  in housing, 77–79, 80–81
  in paint, 77, 82, 151
  in soil, 77, 82

Lead Paint Poisoning Prevention Program, 80, 151
Lead poisoning, 76–83, 151
Legislation
  regarding child battering, 63
  federal, of the 1960s, 2–3, 13, 20–21 (*See also* Community health centers; EPSDT; Hyde Amendment; Lead Paint Poisoning Prevention Program; Maternity and Infant Care projects; Medicaid; WIC)
  regarding lead poisoning, 77–78, 80
  state
    regarding abortions, 40–41
    regarding contraception, 40–41
Low birth weight, 24–36, 145, 147, 148
  abortion and, 29–30
  correlates of, 24
  impact of, 24
  mortality associated with, 9, 16, 21
  poverty and, 24
  screening for anemia in infants of, 91
  in teenagers, 32, 37
  trends in, 25
Low income. *See* Income, low

Marital status. *See* Illegitimacy
Maternity and Infant Care (MIC) projects, 13–14, 26–27, 30–31, 32, 152
MDs. *See* Physicians
Measles, 48, 54–56
Medicaid, 13, 113, 147, 152–53
  coverage of
    for diabetes, 99
    for neonatal intensive care, 17
    for prenatal care, 14–15
  in prevention of lead poisoning, 81
  in teenage childbearing, 39, 40
Medical expenditures, public, 15, 22, 54–56, 73–74, 149, 154
Medical resources. *See* Federal programs, impact of; Medical expenditures, public; Physicians; State programs, for diagnostic testing; Targeting of resources
Medication. *See also* Antibiotics
  in asthma, 131, 133
  in epilepsy, 106
Meningitis. *See* Bacterial meningitis
MIC. *See* Maternity and Infant Care projects
Midwives, 12, 36
Misdiagnosis. *See* Diagnosis
Morbidity, classification of, 153–54
Mortality
  in appendicitis, 120, 122–23
  in asthma, 130, 133, 151
  in bacterial meningitis, 109, 112–13, 116–17
  birth weight–specific, 16, 22, 147, 148
  due to communicable disease, 48, 53, 149–50
  in diabetes, 98, 99
  in epilepsy, 103–4, 105
  in gastroenteritis, 136, 138
  infant, 37, 149
  in lead poisoning, 78–79, 151
  neonatal, 9–17, 145, 146, 147–49
  perinatal, 12, 13
  postneonatal, 20–23, 145, 149
  in rheumatic fever, 58
  in teenage births, 37
Motor vehicles, accidental deaths due to, 149
Mumps (pertussis), 48, 54

Neonatal intensive care, 10, 12, 15, 16–17, 147
Neonatal mortality, 9–17, 145, 146, 147–49
Neurologic complications and sequelae in bacterial meningitis, 113–16
Nurse(s)
  midwives, 12, 26
  practitioners, 13, 100
  public health, 78
Nutrition, 20, 24, 147, 148, 153
  advice regarding, 26–27, 31
  in diabetes, 100
  in gastroenteritis, 137
  in lead poisoning, 77
  supplementation of, 27–29, 90–92
Oral rehydration, 137–38, 152
Organization of services, 2, 72, 151,

153. *See also* Group practice, prepaid; Nurse(s), practitioners; Regionalization
Otitis media, 152
Outcomes of care, xv–xvi
Out-of-wedlock births. *See* Illegitimacy

Parental consent, 40–41
Pertussis, 48, 52–53
Pharyngitis, 60
Phenylketonuria, 71–74, 151
Physicians
  presence of, 116
  type of, in prenatal care, 12, 30–31, 32
Physician-population ratio, 14, 15, 22
Poliomyelitis, 48
Pollution. *See* Air pollution; Environment, lead in
Poor-nonpoor disparities. *See* Income, low
Population-based studies, 145–46, 149, 150, 155, 156. *See also* Epidemiologic studies
Postneonatal mortality, 20–23, 145, 149
Poverty, 9, 24. *See also* Income, low
Predictive value, 65
Prenatal care, 12, 13, 15–17, 147–48, 149
  and low birth weight, 25–27, 30–33
  and neonatal mortality, 12–13, 15–16, 17
  and prevention of child battering, 64, 66
  screening in, 25–26
  in teenage pregnancy, 32
Prepaid group practice. *See* Group practice, prepaid
Prevalence, 4. *See also sections in individual chapters*
Public expenditures. *See* Medical expenditures, public

Race, disparities associated with. *See also* Disadvantaged populations
  in health status
    asthma, 130
    bacterial meningitis, 110
    iron-deficiency anemia, 90
    lead poisoning, 76
    low birth weight, 25
    neonatal mortality, 9, 14–15, 17
    postneonatal mortality, 21–22
    rheumatic fever, 62
    teenage childbearing, 39
  receipt of medical care
    abortions, 43–44
    immunization rates, 51
    prenatal care, 30
Regionalization, 15, 147
Regular source of care. *See* Source of care
Regulation relating to lead poisoning, 81–82
Relative risk, 65
Representativeness of clinical studies, 146
  regarding epilepsy, 107
Resources, medical care. *See* Federal programs, impact of; Medical expenditures, public; Physicians; State programs, for diagnostic testing; Targeting of resources
Rheumatic fever, 58–62, 145, 149, 150
Rubella, 48, 53–54
Rubeola, 48, 54–56

School absence, 92, 130, 131, 132
School requirements for immunizations, 50
Screening
  for anemia, 91
  in child abuse, 65
  for congenital conditions, 71–74
  under EPSDT, 152
  for lead poisoning, 79–81, 82
  in prenatal care, 25–26
Seizures, 103–7
  with bacterial meningitis, 111, 115
Sentinel problems, 2
Services, organization of, 2, 72, 151, 153
Small for gestation age. *See* Intrauterine growth retardation
Smoking
  in asthma, 133

Smoking *(continued)*
   and neonatal mortality, 32
   in pregnancy, 26, 29, 32
Social disadvantage, 152. *See also* Disadvantaged populations; Income, low
Sociodemographic characteristics. *See also* Income, low; Race, disparities associated with
   in low birth weight, 24–26
   in neonatal mortality, 12–15
   in postneonatal mortality, 22, 23
Socioeconomic differentials. *See* Disadvantaged populations; Income, low
Socioeconomic status. *See* Income, low; Social disadvantage
Source of care, 131–32, 151
State programs, for diagnostic testing, 73–74. *See also* EPSDT; Legislation; Medicaid
Statistics, community. *See* Population-based studies
Supreme Court decisions, 40, 149

Targeting of resources, 147, 148
Technology, 113, 147, 150, 154–56
   in neonatal care, 13, 15, 17
   in prenatal care, 25–26
Teenage childbearing, 37–44, 148, 149
   impact of, on infant mortality, 37
Teenagers
   immunization rates in, 51–52, 53, 56
   pregnancies in, 9, 37–44

Tetanus, 48
Therapy, inappropriate or inadequate
   in asthma, 132, 133
   in epilepsy, 106
Throat cultures, 59–60, 61
Time trends. *See* Trends
Trends, 3, 145, 153
   in appendicitis, 120–23
   in asthma, 130
   in bacterial meningitis, 112–13
   in child abuse, 63
   in communicable diseases, 48, 149–50
   in diabetes, 97–98
   in gastroenteritis, 137
   in immunization rates, 48–49
   in iron-deficiency anemia, 87, 89, 93
   in lead poisoning, 76, 78, 80, 81–82
   in low birth weight, 25
   in neonatal mortality, 9–12, 14
   in postneonatal mortality, 20–21
   in rheumatic fever, 58
   in teenage pregnancy, 37–40, 44

Unemployment, 63

Vital statistics, importance of, 145, 146

Well-child care, 152
WIC, 28–29, 91–92. *See also* Nutrition, supplementation of

The Johns Hopkins University Press

The Effectiveness of Medical Care

This book was composed in Times Roman text and display type by BG Composition, Inc., from a design by Chris L. Smith. It was printed on S.D. Warren's 50-lb. Sebago Eggshell Cream paper and bound in Kivar 5 by Bookcrafters.